ALSO BY J. L. KING

On the Down Low

COMING UP
from the

The Journey to

Acceptance,

Healing,

and Honest Love

DOWN
LOW

J. L. King
with Courtney Carreras

Crown Publishers
New York

Published in the United States by Crown Publishers, an imprint of the Crown
Publishing Group, a division of Random House, Inc., New York.
www.crownpublishing.com

CROWN is a trademark and the Crown colophon is a registered trademark of
Random House, Inc.

Library of Congress Cataloging-in-Publication Data
King, J. L.
Coming up from the down low: the journey to acceptance, healing, and honest
love / J. L. King with Courtney Carreras.—1st ed.   1. African American bisexual
men—Sexual behavior.   2. Man-woman relationships.   3. Adultery.   I. Carreras,
Courtney.   II. Title.
HQ74.2.U5K54   2005
305.38'896073—dc22   2005001096

ISBN 1-4000-9846-7

Printed in the United States of America

10   9   8   7   6   5   4   3   2   1

First Edition

I dedicate this book to the memory of my departed mother, Mrs. Lillie Mae King. You were the woman in my life who understood me before I understood myself, and you still loved me.

This book is also dedicated to the many men and women who are seeking relationships based on honesty. I pray that this book is used as a guide to getting past issues that cause people to not be who they are, and allow them to step out of the fog of denial into the light of acceptance.

CONTENTS

CONTENTS

COMING UP
from the
DOWN
LOW

INTRODUCTION

H ello, from Mr. Down Low. That's who I've become over the last year, for better or worse, since the publication of my first book, *On the Down Low: A Journey into the Lives of Straight Black Men Who Sleep with Men.* People yell it out to me in the streets and in airports and in packed elevators, sometimes with affection, sometimes with scorn, sometimes with playful curiosity, and sometimes almost as a threat—"Hey, Mr. Down Low!"

On the Down Low was a blessing and a curse: It brought unprecedented exposure to a topic I consider to be of urgent importance to our community—the hidden lives of black men who sleep with other men while in every other way leading a "straight" life. And it reached a much wider audience than anyone—well, almost anyone—expected. It was a national bestseller that spent more than twenty-six weeks on the *New York Times* bestseller list and became the fuel for a raging debate that went from beauty parlors and barber-shops to the pages of *People* magazine and the soundstage of *The Oprah Winfrey Show.*

And like most raging fires, that debate has grown completely out of control. The interest I hoped to provoke with that first book has turned into a frenzy of speculation, paranoia, and witch-hunting. And while I've been living in the swirl of that frenzy, I've also been deeply affected by it. After all, I primarily used the example of my own life—my own secrets, lies, and eventual transformation—to throw light on the subject, so it was hard to separate the book from my own identity. So I became *Mr. Down Low.*

In the midst of all the excitement and controversy, something else happened. I started to go through some dramatic changes of my own. The experiences of the past year since that first book came out have led me to a new understanding of the down-low phenomenon, and a new understanding of my own life and sexual identity.

I'm a bisexual man. Making this statement is about as hard a thing as I've ever done. Recognizing and accepting this fact about my own identity has been one of the most profound new insights that this year has brought for me. In my first book, I described myself as a straight man who could find sexual gratification with both men and women, but I also claimed that in my heart I could only find true love with a woman. At this point in my journey, it's become clear that it's not that simple for me—or for the many men who are emerging from down-low lives and trying to embrace honesty. I realize now that the same shame and self-deception that sustained my down-low life for so many years was also behind my refusal to entertain the possibility of true intimacy with a man. But now that I've opened myself up to a more complete and honest understanding of myself—helped by listening to the hundreds of men and women I've met over the last few years who are struggling with these same issues themselves—I've come to this liberating truth: I'm not a straight man who has sex with men; I'm a bisexual man. But none of these labels—gay, straight, bisexual—tells my whole story.

That's the most dramatic and personal revelation of the past year or so for me; but I've learned so much more about this phenomenon, its sources, and its consequences. Finally cracking open the down-low phenomenon and letting light flood in has not just driven me to dive deeper into myself, but has created a forum for the thousands and thousands of other people. These are the men and women—straight, gay, and bi—who've been struggling with untold drama in their own lives, but in secret, too ashamed to break their tormented silence. Now these voices have emerged—confused, angry, paranoid, hurt, vengeful, or forgiving, and all too painfully human. We've gone on this journey to deeper understanding together—and not without some bumps in the road.

As I traveled around the country talking about my

book, I was met with more confusion and shock than I would have previously imagined. The most common reactions I found were genuine anxiety and persistent denial that what I was saying was true. Even women who have witnessed down-low behavior first-hand often seemed to be in denial about it—a denial rooted in the pain and betrayal they felt. *How can my husband of twelve years and the father of my two children be gay? . . . My boyfriend is not feminine and always satisfies me in bed, but I think he's sleeping with other men, what's wrong with me? Don't I turn him on? . . . I have never had a problem turning my husband on and he's definitely manly—so even if he has slept with a man, I know that he won't do it again and we can just pray and get through it together.*

I also found unease, to say the least, among women who suddenly started asking uncomfortable questions about the men in their lives. In these women I sometimes saw a fear that bordered on panic and paranoia—these were women who were afraid that the men they loved were harboring secret sexual lives, a fear that in many cases wasn't backed by any actual evidence.

But the saddest responses I ran across came from women, primarily black women, who were still out there looking for the black man of their dreams. The women still searching for The One, the responsible, honest, faithful man who would love and honor them the way they knew they deserved to be loved and honored. These women greeted news about the down low with something like true despair.

Ladies, I hear you. I hear all of you when you express your feelings on the topic. I hear that you are confused, uninformed, and most of all scared about what you're hearing. You are scared for your future and the future of the people you care for.

I clearly remember one woman I met at one of my events. At the end of my presentation, she stood in line with all the others who wanted to get their books signed, but she had another reason for wanting to meet me: She wanted to vent. "I am mad as hell at black men!" is what this beautiful sister said to me. She told me she was giving up on finding a black man who was not gay, not DL, not on drugs, had no criminal record, had a job, and no baby mama drama. This sister told me that she owned her home, had good credit, no children, two degrees, a luxury car, attended church, gave back to her community, was a Big Sister to two inner-city girls, and had not been on a date in over a year.

"Why are brothers doing this to us?" she asked. "Why are black men taking us through this? Why is it that on top of every other problem we have with our men, sisters now have to deal with this down-low *bs*?" She was angry, scared, and confused. As she continued to let loose on me, tears started to well up in her eyes and fall, slowly at first, but soon she was sobbing hard. At this point, I stopped being an author and activist and became a father. She wanted and needed me to tell her everything was going to be okay. As I pulled her to me, to give her a hug and a shoulder to cry on,

I thought about my own daughter who could just as easily be asking me these same questions with the same urgent need for reassurance. This was a sister who did all the right things to be a *queen* for her *king* but still couldn't find a suitable match. As we stood in the middle of the room and I hugged her tightly, I felt myself getting angry at DL men, but not just them. No, my rage started burning at all men who were lying to their women, men who would not commit to relationships, black men who were only dating white women and looking past beautiful sisters. Black men who were locked up, who were strung out on drugs, who were not taking care of their children, who were killing each other in the streets, or who were simply not *showing up*. And the black man that I was most mad at was *me*. I hated myself for all the drama that I had given to all the women who had been in my life. I hated myself for deceiving women who had given me their love, their commitment, their bodies, and most important their trust. I hated myself for all the sisters I took advantage of because of my own selfish needs, who I lured into my web of lies and denial.

I also hated myself when I thought about the sexual relationships that I had with men while in committed relationships with women who believed me when I told them that I loved them and wanted to spend the rest of my life with them. I thought of all the fine sisters who were proud to call me their man, and bragged to their girlfriends and family members that God had sent them the man of their dreams, while all the while I'm living on the DL, lying, sneaking, living undercover, covering up my "other life." I hated what *I used to be.*

As this sister cried on my shoulder, I wanted to cry with her and for her. I wanted her to let *me* cry on *her* shoulder and tell her how sorry I was for the way so many of us had been treating sisters. Then I wanted to cry for all the sisters who were in still in relationships with men on the DL without even knowing it. I was feeling the weight of this sister's pain.

There's enough pain in this to go around. Today with so much attention being put on the DL, many sisters are running for cover. Many are questioning every man in their lives about his sexual history, desires, behaviors, and needs, trying to unearth a secret life. Some are skipping the detective work and just out and out confronting their men with the direct question: "Are you gay?" Brothers from all over the country have asked me to remind sisters that not all black men are on the DL. Many have complained that sisters read my book as the gospel truth about every black man, and now these men are being unjustly accused of being on the DL. They're being accused if they hang out too long with their male friends, if they get a manicure, if they don't answer ringing cell phones. One brother was so pissed off at me for writing my book that he accused me of setting relationships between black men and women back millions of years and told me that because of me, women would probably never trust black men again. One man even threatened me physically at a book fair because he thought my book had caused his girl to turn on him.

The fact is that I am a black man. But the other truth is that I do not speak for or represent *all* black men. When I first spoke openly about my DL lifestyle I was initially speaking to my black community—I felt like I was telling home truths to people who would accept what I had to say because they'd see that I was speaking from the inside, out of knowledge and affection. I was talking about a distinct subculture of black men, not trying to profile all brothers as potentially being on the down low. And I wasn't trying to capitalize on fear or whip up anxiety—I was trying to provide information that would help people make choices based on real information, choices that would help them avoid the heartache and pain I see in my travels all around the country.

To be honest, I'm *stunned* when critics try to act as if I've made this whole phenomenon up out of my own vivid imagination. I only wish that was the case. But the plain and obvious—if painful—truth is this: The down-low phenomenon is real. It's affecting our friends, families, coworkers, fraternity brothers and sorority sisters, and maybe you, the reader, at this very moment. It's breaking hearts, dividing families, and destroying lives. The more information we have, the better we're able to address the problem.

I also thought my message would ring true because I am myself no longer living my life on the down low. Instead of being the problem, I felt that I was truly trying to become part of the solution. I found the strength through prayer to come forward and expose this phenomenon, even if it meant exposing my own dirty laundry in the process. I thought all of this would make my good intentions clear. And despite all of the controversy and distress, the fact is, if I had to do it all over again, I would. Even with the backlash that's come my way because of telling my story, I know that by stepping out I have saved lives. Whenever I read an e-mail from a sister or brother telling me her or his story of emerging from a destructive life of lies, I know that I did the right thing.

But to all the non-DL brothers who feel unfairly accused by the women in their lives, my message to you is this: You need to understand the fear and just deal with it. If you are not guilty and have nothing to hide, then simply step up and tell your woman what she needs to hear. Reassure her that she has nothing to worry about. I know it's not easy to have your sexuality challenged by your woman, but if reassuring her is the price you have to pay to make her feel safe and secure, then I'm sure you'd agree it's worth it.

We are living in a time where it has been documented by the Centers for Disease Control (CDC) that 72 percent of all new HIV infections are happening to black women. That alarming number is evidence that there are some problems in our community when it comes to sex and honesty. Many of these women lived with HIV for months or even longer without even knowing it until they visited a doctor for a routine checkup or because they were pregnant. Many are sisters who were having sex only with their husbands or boyfriends and assumed that their men were having sex only with them. These are women who would never have imagined that their men were having sex outside of their relationships—with women or men.

I hope one day there will be a cure for AIDS. I pray one day that DL men will come up from the down low and be honest and open about their sexual desires and give women a choice to decide their own destiny. But until that day comes, we all have to become more aggressively responsible about our sexual choices to ensure that we live healthy, long lives. If that means some feelings have to get hurt along the way, I'm afraid that's the way it has to be.

It was my interest in HIV education that drove me to write my first book, but in the time I've spent talking about these issues with people all over the country, I've discovered that health issues are just one avenue for confusion and misinformation in our communities. There is also a deep confusion in the culture about sexuality, sexual identity, and the labels we use to identify ourselves.

I found out that many people still don't understand— or don't accept—that people are born with innate sexual preferences. Even in the 2004 presidential debates, the moderator asked the two presidential candidates if they felt homosexuality was a learned behavior or an inherited one. So this question is on the minds of everyone, and, of course, no one *really* has the answer.

But lots of folks still insist that homosexuality is a learned behavior or habit that can be stopped at will—a choice. Whenever I hear this, I have to laugh. *Why*, I think to myself, *would anyone choose this?* Over the course of my life, I've done everything I could to try to make feelings of same-sex attraction go way so that I could just lead the same kind of "straight" life as everyone else, the kind of life that would make it easy for me to fit in with my community and family and just live at peace. But I never could. My sexual desires didn't come from a choice I was making. It was simply who I was.

But still people are confused about how much a person can "control" their sexuality, which has led many men—backed up by the women who love them—to insist that they can become heterosexual through strength of will, even as their bodies and minds rebel against it. I've been in small-town churches where pastors are running programs to "convert" men of questionable sexuality back to the literal straight and narrow and then marry them off—as if laying hands and praying will make a man who has sex with men (MSM) into a heterosexual! This is crazy and just asking for trouble down the road. A person can call himself whatever he wants, but nature is going to find its way, and when it does, all hell will break loose. You can lead a horse to water, as the saying goes. . . .

But all of this just underscores the need for a clearer understanding about sexual behavior and orientation. When I listen to people's questions at my speaking engagements, it's become pretty clear that there is specifically a need for understanding the differences between sexual orientation, identity, and behavior. The fact is that while sexual orientation is something that we're all likely born with, our sexual behavior—including the dangerous, dysfunctional ways we sometimes succumb to our desires, such as when men go on the DL—is something that we can, and must, control.

There is a healing that now has to take place. There is an absolute need for more specific information about the DL lifestyle that will help end this epidemic and change the way people live and love. This book intends to shed some of that light. I wrote *On the Down Low* because it was necessary. Necessary, first of all, to create a platform for discussion. Without open communication and the ability to recognize our choices we are all at risk. And I wrote this new book because people still want to know more. They want to know *why* this is happening, *where* this is happening, and *how* the healing can begin. I also wrote this book to show that I have changed and no longer live my life on the DL and that other men are capable of change as well.

People always ask me: what makes me an authority on all of this? Am I a physician or a mental health professional? Am I an expert on sex and relationships? Well, the truth is that I'm none of those things. But I've done a lot of research, starting with the most expensive kind of research there is: personal experience. But I knew my personal experience wasn't enough. I wanted to get other DL men's opinions on how they felt about living undercover. I wanted to ask them if they felt the same way I did, and how they dealt with the guilt from their double lives (or if they even felt guilty at all). I wanted to know that I was not alone. I had many friends who were on the DL and they knew still more men on the DL, which provided me with my first pool of anecdotal research. We would get together and tell stories about ourselves and the men we had been with sexually. We would share "war stories" about the brother who was married, or the one who was a pastor, or the deep undercover brother who no one would ever suspect of messing around with other men. This was fascinating—and enlightening—but now I wanted to know even more. So I started reaching out to brothers all over the country. I placed ads on popular sex websites. I met brothers at various churches I'd visit and tapped into my network of friends in all the major cities around the country who would each hook me up with a DL bro to talk to. I also would go to popular cruising sites and pick up brothers with the intent to discover their stories. And because I worked in the state of Ohio prison system with thousands of men, I contacted brothers who were locked up and living DL lives.

Then I received a contract from the Ohio Department of Health/HIV office to conduct a survey of DL men in five Ohio cities. This process allowed me to talk to many more men who volunteered to share their stories of sex and lies.

I also dug through my past for clues that would help put together the larger picture of the DL phenomenon. I thought back to my eight years in the United States Air Force and the many men I met while stationed at bases and overseas with whom I had sex. I remembered the time when I was stationed in San Antonio, where there were lots of military men stationed, both Army and Air Force. I was still well connected with them and knew that for certain brothers in uniform, sexual hookups were the norm. And these were men who were bound by the rules of the military to live straight lives.

While I was doing my research on my first book, I would spend days just responding to personal ads on the top five DL websites. Sometimes I would be up all night in online chat rooms with names like "For DL Brothers Only." Before I knew it, I was hooked on connecting with men all over the world through web cameras. It wasn't just me; my best friend would sit in front of his PC for hours looking at other men around the country who would masturbate and do sexual acts for others to watch . . . the wonderful world of the net will bring whatever you need to you without ever leaving the comforts of your home.

Although my first impulse was to do research to get to the bottom of this phenomenon, the truth is that all this "research"—visiting men on the DL underground, checking out the websites, answering personals—only fed my addiction to sex with men. I was definitely learning things about

these men's lives and was trying to keep it strictly informa-
tional, but, next thing you know, I was making quick
hookups to satisfy my own lusts and desires. The conversations would take a sharp turn from interviews to seductions;
the email exchanges got faster and more intensely sexual. I
got caught up and before I knew it, I was deep back into a
sexually risky and dishonest space—even though I kept lying
to myself about the "research."

Eventually I came to grips with it and realized I needed
to get a handle on this addiction. Once I honestly dealt
with the reality that I was out of control, I was able to break
away and get refocused. But the fact is, even when the research turned into "research," it gave me valid and intimate
insights into the phenomenon and into my own case in
particular.

All this experience is what I brought to my books and
to my audience in a raw and direct way. This openness is one
reason that for every person who listens intently to my message there's another person who fears it. For many people, I
am the first black man they've encountered who has ever
openly talked about his sexual history with other men.

So when I wrote that first book, I wanted to use my life,
my research, and my opinions to show the dangers of this
behavior and provide answers and information to educate
all parties affected by the DL lifestyle. My goal was not to
place another negative stigma on black men; it was to educate and draw awareness about a behavior that was destructive

to our community. And to be honest with you, I was going into this blind. I did not foresee that I would be receiving all this media exposure. I just wanted to tell my story, hoping it would provide some new information for those who researched the spread of HIV. And in turn I encouraged them to get this information to those who needed to know it, including my own daughter.

You see, when I wrote that book, I was also thinking as a father. I wanted all fathers to walk in my shoes to understand why I did this, why I came out, why I do what I do. All I had to do was to look at my daughter and other beautiful women who were being lied to. All I had to do was read an e-mail, or have a conversation with a woman who has been infected by her man. All I have to do is talk to a DL friend of mine who is still living his life as if he is some invincible superhuman, knowing that he has a wife who doesn't know about his bisexuality. I asked the fathers, brothers, uncles, and male friends who are on the DL to come forward for the women in their lives. I asked them to understand why I have. Would you want your daughter, sister, niece, or girlfriend to be involved with a man who is lying to her, especially about his sexual behavior? No man should inflict the type of pain that comes from this deceptive behavior.

My message was that the man on the DL needs to take a close look at himself. He needs to ask himself if he has the right to play God, if he has the right to put the person he is intimate with in danger of emotional damage and health-related problems. This was the struggle I went through in my own life and this was my motivation in writing that first book.

One month prior to the book being released I got a call from *The Oprah Winfrey Show* producers. In the book world this is good for business, but in my world it was a blessing. This call changed my life forever.

While I was sitting on Oprah's couch less than two feet from her, she turned to me and told me that when she picked up my book she couldn't put it down. Oprah understood the importance of my message and was right there helping me get the word out to the people. It was unbelievable to me to see how encouraging she was. She called the book revealing and courageous. I thank her for that. I thank her for reminding me that although I have hurt others in the past with this behavior, I can now help to break that cycle.

This book in part is the story of the evolution of my own understanding of this phenomenon. I started out on this path thinking in terms of HIV/AIDS, but I came to realize that the down-low phenomenon is not just a public-health issue, but a symptom of a much broader issue in our community. It's about relationships and how we think about sex and love and honesty.

Over the last few years, I've encountered thousands of people who are dealing with these issues every day of their lives, people who've come up to me after my presentations or written to me after they've read my book and opened

COMING UP FROM THE DOWN LOW

their hearts, telling me about the secrets they've harbored and the feelings they've struggled with, but also about the many ways they've found healing, hope, and resolution. These people have given me a kaleidoscopic view of this phenomenon, from every imaginable perspective. In other words, when I talk about these issues, I'm not speaking from a book or a study, I'm speaking from the flesh-and-blood-and-tears experiences of your family, friends, and neighbors, your classmates and fellow parishioners who've struggled with this and, in some cases, triumphed.

And, of course, I'm also talking about my own life. I've *lived* this and been struggling down the road of understanding my entire life. Since the publication of the first book I've made further progress down that road, helped along by the thousands of you who responded. The insights I've gotten have transformed my understanding of this phenomenon and transformed my life. I want to share those insights with you now, to help you better understand the down-low phenomenon, yes, but also to help you better understand the potential liberating power of honesty, acceptance, and healing in our personal lives and in the life of our community.

The rewards for spreading the word have been many. Women come up to me all the time to tell me that they are now set free. They thought that they were losing their minds when they went through their own DL experience, but now they know they're not alone and have the courage to act. I also encounter many DL brothers who are really looking at themselves and making a conscious effort to change, to become more sexually responsible. I also have found a way to talk openly and honestly with my daughter about my life. To share the truth. That I can say is one of the biggest blessings from this entire experience.

Now, let the journey continue . . .

THE CYCLE

Early last year, my photo appeared on the cover of *Jet* magazine. I was wearing a slick black designer suit over an open-collared white shirt—the photo was serious, sexy, and undeniably masculine. As a black man who came of age in the 1960s and 70s, appearing on the cover of the legendary *Jet* magazine was an important signifier that I'd made it. To me, *Jet* is still the final word on who's who in the black community. But it was even more important than that to me. You see, one of the great fears of every man or woman who hides the truth about their sexuality is that as soon as they're exposed, they'll be cast out of the community, exiled for breaking the rules. For me, that fear was multiplied many times over. When I published my first book, which revealed my own complicated sexual life in detail, I wasn't just exposing myself to my immediate friends and family, but I was bascially stripping myself naked in front of the entire community. If I was going to be rejected and cast out for what I revealed about myself, there was no place for me to turn.

Which brings me back to that *Jet* magazine cover. When I got that first copy of the magazine in my hands, my heart swelled—not just with pride, but with relief. I saw in it an affirmation that people—my *own* people—understood and respected what I was doing and still embraced me. I blew that photo up into a giant poster and hung it in my office. It's there now, the first thing any visitor sees.

But the next day, I got a rude awakening when I turned on my radio to listen to the *Tom Joyner Morning Show*. Tom Joyner's radio show is like the electronic equivalent of *Jet* magazine; it's the most popular radio show among black people around the country, with a national audience in the millions. I tuned into the show to hear Joyner and his comedian sidekick, J. Anthony Brown, *howling* about the *Jet* photograph. They were straight clowning me, talking about how gay I looked and how only a dummy would ever believe that I could pass myself off as straight. I was deeply embarrassed. They went on and on to the point where I decided to go back and look at the magazine myself. By now, I was embarrassed to even pick up the magazine again. For the photo to become such a big joke, I figured it must be pretty bad. Eventually I picked up the magazine and checked out the photo again. Yep, there I was, just as I remembered, staring back at the camera, my features set, my posture rigid, my clothing perfectly stylish but by no means effeminate.

I started wondering why Joyner and his morning show crew seemed to be pushing their joke so hard. But then it suddenly came to me. Let me explain: In traditional black male culture, we're taught from a young age to fear the sissy, the freak, the faggot. But we're also taught that it's easy to pick one out of a crowd, which is why as a man, you're taught to be very careful about the signals you give off. For instance, when I was a kid, if my father caught me crossing my legs a certain way when I sat down, he'd rush over and push my knees apart to make sure my feet were planted firmly on the ground. "Never cross your legs like that—that's how women sit," he'd tell me. *Really?* I clearly wasn't a woman, I was a little boy, but the unspoken message in my father's words was that appearances count—to appear less than manly was to *be* less than manly. But he also implied that the reverse was true: if you *acted* manly, it meant you were fully a man—a heterosexual man. So, he seemed to say, if I only sat the right way, everything would be okay.

But that's why the idea of the down low threw so many black men for a loop. Here I am, someone who spent time in the military, had a wife and kids, attended church every Sunday, sexed more women than a lot of guys could imagine, and now I'm telling you that I have sex with men. It doesn't make sense to traditional-minded men (or women, for that matter). More than that, it scares them. It means that what they've been taught about identifying sexuality is not necessarily true. It means that sexuality is looser and harder to define than they ever allowed themselves to imagine. It means that no matter how a man crosses his legs, you still don't know who he's fucking when the lights go out and the shades are drawn. That's a threat to people who cling to more traditional ideas about sexual identity and orientation. And the response to that threat is often vicious homophobia. Rather than try to make sense of the complicated reality about sexuality, which is that people get down in thousands of different variations, not just "gay" and "straight," some people will try to attack and banish whatever it is they don't understand. They try to exile the bisexual, or the gay brother or sister, or the brother struggling to come up from the down low, thinking that by making these confusing people invisible, it will somehow put their own minds back at ease. They're wrong.

So that's why some of my critics do their best to categorize me as gay. I've often wondered where this need for labels comes from. For some people, it's a defense mechanism, a way to strip away whatever masculinity I have and send me off, so they can relax again. That's nothing new. For many men who live in traditional black communities, the word *gay* is a loaded term, often used as a weapon. It's name-calling and has the same effect as it does in the schoolyard when the guys circle around and start snapping on the fat kid or the skinny kid or the kid with the played-out clothes. The purpose is to intimidate and to silence and to divide, to create an us-against-them mentality.

After being so happy about feeling the embrace of the community by being on the cover of *Jet,* it was a fast turn-around to feel ridiculed on the *Tom Joyner Show*. Of course, everybody knows that Tom Joyner and his crew talk about everyone, and in our community everyone is fair game for the "dozens," so there's no point in taking it personally. And Tom has since then supported me and my work by having me on his HBCU cruise. Even with his jokes, the fact that he mentioned me and my book on his show helped me get the word out. So I have nothing but respect for the man and the positive work he does in the community. Still, I'm only human.

But this low point became a key for me. It helped clarify one of the reasons men go on the down low rather than simply identifying themselves as gay or bisexual and calling it a day. No one wants to be ostracized and excommunicated from the world they know and love. No one wants to lose a place in the culture that sustains them. And no one wants to be the kid in the schoolyard again, being dissed and snapped on until he's forced to find a lonely corner by himself. Labels do count.

I have been asked many times what exactly "on the down low" really means. My answer has never changed. The *down low*, or *DL*, generally refers to the lifestyle of black men who consider themselves heterosexual and live publicly heterosexual lives—even to the point of being married to women, in some cases—but who also have sex with men without telling their female partners.

I've also been asked many times if I am the creator of the term "down low." Of course the answer to that is no. The term was originally devised to describe any kind of slick, secretive behavior, including infidelity in heterosexual relationships. The term has been common in the lyrics of many R&B songs. Singer R. Kelly made the phrase famous in his song "Down Low (Nobody Has to Know)": *We can keep it on the down low / Nobody has to know.* That song (and the video that went with it) was all about heterosexual infidelity. But the term was eventually adopted by the subculture of men who lead "straight" lives but sleep with other men on the side.

The subtitle of my first book was *A Journey into the Lives of "Straight" Black Men Who Sleep with Men.* This not only raised a lot of eyebrows, it raised a lot of questions: How can you say that sex between a man and another man is not gay? Are you saying that a man who has sex with another man but is married to a woman is still straight? What's the difference between a man on the down low and a bisexual man who practices both hetero and homosexual sex? Aren't down-low men just gay men trying to have it both ways?

The mistake in all of those questions is that people confuse what *they* want to call these men with what these men want to call themselves. Let me explain: If you're a bisexual man who doesn't want anyone to know you're bisexual, you'll simply call yourself straight. If you're a closeted gay man, you'll tell all the world that you're straight. Anyone with any sense knows that a man who is regularly having sex with another man is not straight by any conventional definition of the word. But we used that subtitle to make a very important point: despite their sexual lives and preferences, many DL men consider themselves to be straight because that's the face they put on for the world. This is one of the fundamental features of the DL man. He doesn't necessarily think that his sexual behavior—having sex with men—changes his identity as a straight man. He doesn't want what happens in his sexual life to in any way conflict with the entitlements that go to straight men in the world: a wife, a traditional family, and a secure place in the community.

Like many slang terms, DL means different things to different people. There are many variations of DL brothers. Some DL men identify themselves as straight, have wives and girlfriends, but also secretly have sex with other men. Others on the DL are younger men who are still questioning or exploring their sexuality, but are not comfortable yet in claiming a same-gender-loving (SGL) identity, so they keep their sexual identity on the down low. Some DL men are closeted gay or bisexual men—men who acknowledge their gay or bisexual identities to themselves, but who are not open about it. These men may exclusively have sex with other men, or with both men and women, but because of the stigma placed on gay people, they stay closeted.

The common denominator is that a person on the DL stays on the DL for fear of the backlash that outing himself will bring on. This is especially true in the African American community, where even a man who claims that he's bisexual is still only seen as gay. And gay in our community usually means *faggot, sissy, queer.* The lack of acceptance of the gay *masculine* man in the African American community has led many gay or bisexual men to live their lives on the DL. These men are unwilling or afraid to be labeled by the stereotypes that society and the media have placed on anything attached to the word *gay.* These men don't want to have their lives turned into some *Will and Grace* stereotype—they're not dressing like the men on *Queer Eye for the Straight Guy* or hanging out at the "Birdcage." In other words, they have difficulty accepting the whole package of the gay *lifestyle.* And, in many cases, their own sexuality is not simply a matter of preferring men over women—they actually like both. For these men sexuality is a not an item on a menu, but a long, varied buffet they want to pick and choose from. More important, they don't think that the way they behave in their sexual lives should have any impact on the rest of their lives—they don't think sex is the thing that defines them. So rather than come out and let people label them in a restrictive way, they create a secret life for themselves where they can practice their sexual preferences as they choose, while still maintaining a straight identity to the public. They start living their lives on the DL.

This complexity about labels and identity extends to black men who are already out of the closet and living openly gay lives, who still reject obvious, flamboyant displays of their orientation and even reject using the word *gay*. Black men who reject the labels of *gay* or *bisexual* have received negative criticism from the white gay community. If you talk to many African American gay community leaders, they will tell you that this tension is growing.

I have been told by many of my gay friends that the tension stems from the lack of support the African American gay community shows to the gay movement as a whole. Some claim that while the white gay community is extremely open about their fight to be accepted and have equal rights, the black gay community has not joined that struggle, yet still benefits from the progress the movement has brought. Some in the white gay community feel that black gay men need to join the fight.

Many of the African American homosexual friends I have object to the idea that they have to adopt the same tactics as the white gay community. They feel that their fight has to be waged internally, inside our own community, before we can begin to make any efforts outside. This isn't to say that there are *no* black men who have taken up the cause of gay rights. There are African American gay men who stand shoulder to shoulder with their white gay counterparts and joined them in the fight for equal rights and for equality in general. There is an organization headed by an outspoken black gay activist that is on the front lines of gay rights. But I recently said in an interview that many of my gay friends find that they cannot be both black and gay in their community and still find acceptance. This activist disagreed and claimed that there are many out and proud black gay men who feel comfortable being black and gay in their 'hood. I don't know about that. When I asked my gay friends if they feel like they can be out, gay, and proud in their hometowns and communities, not one of them said yes. I personally don't know many men who are willing to hang a gay flag on their porch or even hold hands going in or out of their worship service. And I am still waiting to meet an *out* gay couple to come forward and tell the world that they are active in their fraternity. Most of my gay friends are still very much deep in the closet. This is the tension that sometimes erupts in DL behavior.

I recently had a conversation with an associate who is gay. I asked him if he was willing to allow me to tell people that he is gay, and he said, "Hell no, what I do in my bedroom is my business." I find this attitude to be more common than not.

This tension about sexuality and privacy is obviously linked to the mentality of DL men, who take it one step further by keeping their sexual lives secret even from those with whom they're intimate: their friends, families, and lovers. In fact, as shocking as it may seem, I discovered that the DL term is used by some men as a label of pride. To these men, saying they are on the DL is showing that they are undetectable and capable of getting away with secret sexual behavior. I personally have gay friends who *prefer* to keep their status on the DL. To them that means they can attract more men or the kind of masculine men who don't want to be associated with "out" gay men.

The differences among the white and black communities extend to the language they use to describe themselves. I have a very close African American friend who absolutely considers himself homosexual. He in no way pretends to be straight, bisexual, or anything else other than gay. However, like a lot of African American gay men, he chooses to use the term *SGL,* or "same gender loving," when describing his sexual orientation, instead of *gay,* because he believes that *gay* has come to be associated with a certain kind of white homosexual.

My friend Frank, who considers himself to be a "hands-on" activist for gay rights, refuses to participate in any activities planned by the white gay community. When he is asked to be part of a march for gay marriages, or demonstrate for anything that his white gay counterparts are trying to secure, he declines. He is active at his church and has established an SGL ministry with the support of his pastor. He mentors young gay men and hosts presentations about HIV education as well as fundraisers to support programs that work with HIV/AIDS individuals. Frank has also mentored many gay men—both adults and youth—who are coming out and trying to understand what being "in the life" means. He also works with parents who know that their children are homosexual. Frank is doing his part. To him, being in front of television cameras or giving radio interviews and locking arms with white gay men marching down a street is not how he wants to make change. He believes that in his community there is a better, more effective way to make change happen without pushing or forcing sexuality on the people. He doesn't want to have to deal with the stares, gossip, and finger pointing that he would get from black folks to whom homosexuality is still taboo, no matter how much we might wish it otherwise. So while he works hard *within* the community to help other black gay men in a variety of ways, he's not going to march down Main Street flying the flag with a line of white gay men.

He once told me that he hosted a cookout at his house and invited many of his black and white gay friends. His black gay friends had been to his house before and knew that coming to his house required keeping one's sexuality on the DL. Not that they had anything to hide, but they were not going to walk up to his house holding hands. He assumed that his white gay friends would practice the same discretion. He lives in a very urban neighborhood that has not yet embraced the "gay next-door neighbor."

Toward the end of the evening, someone suggested that when the guests were leaving to go home, they remain discreet and not call attention to themselves while walking down the street to their cars. My friend, the party host, agreed. He was aware that the brothers and sisters that hang out near the corners and or sit on their porches all night were not necessarily gay friendly, and he didn't want his guests to be harassed.

But one of the white gay guests got upset with this suggestion and protested that he would not hide who he is, and that he would walk right down the middle of the block holding his lover's hand if he wanted to and wouldn't give a damn what anyone had to say about it.

This comment launched a huge debate about the balance between personal integrity and community acceptance. One of the more outspoken white guests said, "Black gay men need to just be who they are, quit lying to everyone about who they are, and start living their lives as open and proud gay men." He accused his black gay friends of being just as homophobic as heterosexuals who reject the gay community as a whole. To many of the black men in the room, this accusation was preposterous. To them, it was less important to push their gay identity than it was to retain a place in the black community. To openly and aggressively embrace a "gay" identity, to many of these black men, was to turn their back on the larger black community that sustained them. The outspoken white gay man just didn't understand this difficult balancing act—instead, he just hurled out an uninformed accusation.

It's just that type of comment that has caused many black gay men to drop the label *gay* altogether when describing themselves. It's this kind of perceived ultimatum—*you have to make a choice to be black or to be gay, to link arms with the black community or with the (predominantly white) gay community*–that has breathed life into the DL behavior. For some black men, DL life is the only way that they can live their lives with real sexual freedom, while also being loyal to the larger community of black people. Most black men do not want to be associated with the standards and manner of self-definition that most white gay men subscribe to. And they fear being tarred with the stereotypes of white gay behavior. This conflict in the minds of black gay men is one of the defining elements of DL men: trying to find a way to maintain a home in the fraternities, churches, and families that they've had their entire lives and to be open and honest about their sexuality at the same time. This is not to defend the men who choose to go underground with their sexuality, but at the same time it's critical to understand the pressures that drive them there.

There are also variations and differences among men who are on the DL. Just because they share certain elements of the same lifestyle doesn't mean they're all the same. Far from it. Some DL men don't want to associate with other DL men who they feel are too risky with their behavior and leave themselves open to discovery or unsafe sex. I have a friend who feels that he is on a higher level than other DL men because he *ain't no ho*. He told me that he would never cruise a park or adult bookstore to pick up men. That's too trashy for him. He only deals with men who are part of an elite group of professional black men. These men don't have sex outside of their class. They allow other DL men to be a part of their group or brotherhood based on their jobs, looks, homes, and other social and economic classifications that weed out the unworthy. But what most DL men are looking for is an environment where they can finally feel some safety and security, away from the judging eyes of straight people, the pressures of gay activist types, or the risks of less discreet brothers.

I recently attended a party in Miami that was hosted by a very powerful brother who works in law. He wanted me to meet other brothers who, as he stated to me, are "in your class," meaning, brothers who are well-paid, educated, and don't tell one another's business outside of the circle. He told me that these are the type of brothers that I need to associate myself with, not those common brothers who are like messy sissies who tell all your business and use you as they see fit. It's always funny to me that even within this secretive subculture built on dishonest behavior, people seek to set themselves apart from one another, as if there's a "right" way to live a DL life. But on the other hand, I understood this brother's desire to create a safe space.

At the party I met some successful brothers who were from all walks of life: lawyers, doctors, ministers, and businessmen. Many of these men were part of a very closed secret society within the DL community. Not all of the men were bisexual: some of the men there were completely out; others were closeted and on the DL. These men, even though they weren't out, exactly, were comfortable in their skin as gay men in this kind of closed environment, if not in the outside world.

There's something clearly wrong with this kind of party, but at the same time, as Chris Rock would say, *I understand.* Parties like these are safe havens for men who otherwise wouldn't have a place to go—it's something they need. I don't defend the fact that some men on the DL go to parties like this explicitly to find sex partners, which is another way of saying they go to these parties to cheat on the women in their lives with men. At the same time, one could argue that it's better here than at a public park or some other risky, dangerous spot. The thing is, these DL men have built a system of support, which is a completely human reaction to a situation where they'd otherwise be alone. It's hard to fault them for that. They're simply looking for camaraderie. But in spite of my sympathy for these brothers, I know what they're doing is wrong. When I see a high-profile minister hanging out at an exclusive DL party, I know that minister's wife is at home, or at her mama's house, or with her girlfriends, or out with the kids wondering where her man is, maybe even sick to her heart because she suspects the truth. When I see some young, good-looking professional man at the spot, I know there's a good chance he's got a woman somewhere on the side who has no idea about this secret life. I can't defend that. It makes me sick to think about it.

But the problem is not strictly with the DL brother; it's a much larger issue. When people carry on, laughing and poking fun and ostracizing gay and bisexual brothers, they push their behavior underground. It makes me mad that for these DL brothers to experience any sense of comfort or camaraderie at all they have to go creeping off into secrecy, rather than being able to lead their lives in the open, without fear. I know how wonderful it feels for me to be at these kinds of parties now, as opposed to when I was living a secret life. Now, I'm just having a good time, being my natural self. I'm not thinking in the back of my mind about what lie I'm going to have to construct when I get home. When I see brothers sneaking to a quiet spot in the room so they can answer their cell phones and pretend they're somewhere else to the person on the other end, it reminds me of my former life. I know that feeling. I used to spend half my brain cells trying to scheme up ways to cover my tracks when I was living on the DL. Over time, I figured out the tricks of the trade. I'd douse myself with cologne to cover up the smell of sex and remember to come up with elaborate excuses to explain why I put a hundred miles on the car when all I was supposed to be doing was visiting my friend two blocks away. But even the most savvy vet at living down low can slip up. When you're on the down low, you're haunted no matter where you go, even in a supposedly "safe" party.

It all goes back to the larger cycle of fear in our communities. And we all have a part to play in breaking that cycle and freeing ourselves. Brothers on the down low need to take a stand for honesty, even though it's hard. But the rest of us need to make it easier for them to take that stand. We all need to just drop the homophobia and fear that drive men with perfectly normal, natural sexual desires underground, where this behavior becomes dangerous and destructive.

2.

THE REAL ISSUE
IS INFIDELITY

"Ye shall know the truth, and the truth shall make you free."

—John 8:32

A h, if only it were that easy. There are so many reasons why people lie, deceive, and cheat. But let me make a revolutionary statement: Honesty is the basis of healthy relationships, no matter what your sexual orientation is.

Okay, maybe that's not such a revolutionary statement. But it's the kind of plain truth people easily forget. When it comes to our most intimate relationships, infidelity stems from a whole range of things, including the raw need to fulfill a sexual desire—we're all human and sometimes weak. Although people like to hold DL men out for special condemnation, the fact is that cheating is cheating. And as long as we pretend that the only cheating that matters is DL cheating, we're missing the point. The DL phenomenon is happening against the backdrop of a growing culture of cheating and infidelity and uncommitted sex, regardless of sexual orientation.

I recently met a couple at one of my presentations who told me that they have five daughters and none of them is married. Three of the five are still living at home and they are all over thirty years old. The reason this couple was at the presentation was because these five unmarried daughters had produced for them eight granddaughters, so they knew they were sexually active. They just wanted to learn about HIV to make sure their daughters were at least going to be safe. The man told me that none of his daughters had a steady man in their life. He said that most of them had been in very rocky relationships and the men who had fathered their grandchildren were not remotely responsible. Although he came to the presentation looking for guidance on HIV, it turned out that his deeper concern was trying to figure out why his daughters were willing to settle in their relationships and put their lives or their emotions at risk.

This is a question that comes up repeatedly in my presentations. Talking about the DL phenomenon always stirs up a larger question: *Forget about why men go on the DL, tell me why the hell women are willing to settle for these cheating, lying, scheming men?*

During my speaking engagements I feel compelled to

ask a question to my audience: "When did relationships change to where there are so few long-term, happily married couples?" I wonder what's changed from back in the day when our grandparents met and stayed married for what seemed like forever. When I read about couples celebrating their fortieth, fiftieth, or even sixtieth wedding anniversaries, I try to imagine what the key element is to their marriage lasting so long. It seems obvious that their wisdom and experience could be used to help us all create better relationships, ones that are not based on short-term goals.

At one of my presentations, after I went into my ode to the long-term relationships of the past, one woman stood up and responded, "But even back then, were there really as many happy couples as we thought?" She went on to speak about the false impressions and smoke screens people put up and the secrets couples hid away from from friends and family. And she's right. It's naive to idealize the past.

My mother and father were married for more than fifty years before my mom passed away. They stuck together through the good times and the bad. Back then in our small town it was unheard of for a couple to get divorced—no matter what the struggle, the man and woman were expected to work it out somehow. Even when my parents were on nonspeaking terms, my dad always came home after work, and my mother always made sure that dinner was on the table and my father's clothes were clean. I remember hearing them fight about bills or some other minor issue, but at the end of the day my parents were in the same bed together. As a child, it made me feel secure to know that no matter what happened, my parents were going to end the day together. As a community, it made us all feel secure to know that no matter what happened, the families that made up that community would stay intact. But who knows what personal costs all of those parents, all of those husbands and wives, paid to stay together?

Now we have choices that people of that generation lacked—sometimes it seems like we have too many choices, since these choices can cause heartache in others. Just as our parents and grandparents figured out a way to balance their own desires with the need to make sacrifices for their families and communities, we too need to figure out a balance that makes sense for our times. It's not a matter of idealizing the past, or trying to live like we're in the 1950s; the urgent need right now is for us to figure out a healthy, responsible way to live today.

Many DL men have said to me that they wanted to stop cheating on their women. I know one married brother who told me that he had relationships outside of his marriage with both men and women and he was tired of being stretched so thin, but at the same time he was too scared to be honest because he didn't want to lose his family. He told me that if he ever found the strength to open up to his wife, he'd apologize and ask forgiveness. He was even willing to get counseling for his cheating and his "out-of-control sex drive." He told me he loved his wife, and was seeking advice from me on what should he do. I encouraged him to open up and be honest with his woman, but I also told him to be braced for the hurricane of emotion he might get in response. The difficult thing is that just being open and honest doesn't guarantee that your story is going to have a happy ending—it usually only means that you're beginning a new struggle.

But on the flip side, it's important that women who've gone through this as innocent victims try to reach deep inside of themselves to find some compassion if they can. I know it's difficult to forgive someone who has cheated on you and taken advantage of your love and trust, but you can still strive to attain some understanding about why this thing has happened—and to be open to the possibility that the relationship can be saved. I know to a lot of you women out there, this sounds crazy, but let me explain.

Sometimes, the boundaries we create in our own minds stop us from healing. When someone on the DL comes forward, however dark it may initially seem to the one that was deceived, the light will shine. But for most women, they don't even spare a second to consider the possibility of forgiveness. I have encountered several women who've told me flat out, "If my man tells me he is on the DL, I am *leaving* his ass." I was recently in Atlanta speaking to a group when one woman made it clear to the roomful of people that she felt this way, that she would in no way be able to forgive her man. She said she would not only leave him, but probably swear off men forever! If she really did find herself in that situation, I don't know if she would really follow through on that. I hope she never has to find out. The fact is that for women who are confronted with the reality of a down-low lover or spouse, it's always more complicated than it seems. They have to make a decision based on the complicated human being in front of them.

I have heard many women tell me that after they found out that their man was on the DL, it was like the death of a dream. They felt they needed time to mourn and were unsure how they were going to go on, since the foundation of their entire past—the love that was central to their lives—now felt like a lie. Other woman have told me that discovering that a man is on the 'low doesn't put an end to the love they have for that man. These are women who feel that true love is deep enough and real enough to allow them to accept anything.

Now I know some of you out there are snickering or shaking your heads in disbelief that anyone would stick by a DL man. But when I hear women make those kinds of declarations, my mind goes to all the wives and girlfriends that visit men who are incarcerated. These are women who work hard all week and then bring money for their mate's commissary. I think of mothers and wives and girlfriends who take the early bus in the freezing cold and travel long distances to the middle of nowhere, undergo searches and stares and the sadness of standing in the shadow of a penitentiary, just to spend an hour to see men who are locked up for crimes like murder and rape. I'm sure it seems crazy to some folks, but even in these trying situations, there are women who are *committed* to their men and are going to be there for them no matter what.

So I understand when women tell me that they are willing to work it out with a DL man who's trying to do better. This doesn't always mean that these women are willing to continue on in intimate relationships with these men. Many of these women simply commit to maintain close friendships with their spouses so that the children can grow up around a family that is intact, if not in the traditional sense. My relationship with my exwife is a good example of how a couple can heal and move on with their lives. I cheated on her in the worst way. I lied to her and in many ways made a mockery of our vows, all because of my own sexual confusion and out-of-control appetite. She was smart enough to terminate our relationship, and she was also smart enough not to let my confusion stop her from finding love and moving on with her life. She is a strong woman who thought about our children and used every bit of wisdom and resilience she had to keep things together when everybody was telling her that her life was falling apart. She was able to pull it together and move on. She was not going to let me stop her from living. And she wanted me to be involved with our children and even maintained a relationship with my parents, to whom she'd grown close over the years of our marriage.

How one person chooses to deal with it may not be reasonable for another. Each couple is different and there is no telling how they'll react. There are so many factors. For instance, couples share many things in a relationship and sex is only one of them. To some couples the love and companionship they share is the most important element of their relationship and they can stay together without sexual intimacy or even sexual exclusivity.

My friend Chuckie is a very successful businessman who lives in the "Bible Belt"—the Deep South. He was married and had what appeared to be a classic beautiful life: the house, the cars, the successful business, and the beautiful wife. But he wasn't happy. One day he came home and simply came out with it: He told his wife he was gay. Not bisexual, not DL, not curious, but gay. He told me he was tired of living a lie, and was willing to give up the house and cars and give his wife whatever she wanted if she decided to divorce him. He didn't need possessions to make him happy. He just wanted to be free from the guilt and free to be true to himself and to his wife.

But his wife didn't want a divorce, much to his surprise. Initially she was shocked, but she loved him and respected him for telling her about his sexuality, recognizing how hard it was for him, a high-profile, successful black man in a conservative, religious community, to come out. Somehow, this heightened the bond they shared. They worked out their relationship and remained together. Now, the dynamic of their relationship is completely different than what they'd intended when they said their vows more than fourteen years earlier in front of God and their family and friends.

They no longer share a bed. In fact, Chuckie's wife lives in one wing of the house, and he lives in the other. Their young son doesn't know about or fully understand this arrangement yet—as far as he can tell, he's just got two parents living at home, providing him a secure environment. And they both do their best to make sure that he always has a normal life with two loving parents. They will deal with explaining their situation to him as he gets older. To the outside world they appear to be perfectly happy. And the truth is that *they are.* What the world sees is a traditional married couple; what they do in their home is their business. They have not stopped doing anything they did before, except having sex with each other. She was willing to give up sex in their relationship. She even told him that she will not cheat on him, because she vowed in front of her God to be with him only. She has forgiven him for not telling her he was gay from the onset. For his part, he does not bring men home, and he does nothing to disrespect her or their home.

This solution is not for everyone, but it is for Chuckie and his family. It may seem that Chuckie's wife has made an unsustainable bargain or is fooling herself. I don't know the truth of what's going on in either of their hearts. But what I do know is that by coming forward and being honest with his wife, Chuckie gave her a *choice.* You or I may not agree with the choice she's made, but the fact is that she got all any of us can ask for: honest information from which to make important life decisions. I am proud of Chuckie for coming forward and giving his wife the honesty she deserves. And I admire his wife for choosing to support her gay husband and understanding what a hard road this has been for him to travel.

On the opposite end of the spectrum is Willie, a brother in Denver I met recently. He told me that he is okay with his bisexuality and feels that he is not cheating on his wife because he is only having sex with men. He doesn't think it qualifies as cheating as long as he's not emotionally connected to the men he is having sex with. He is always at home with the family and proudly stated that he always practices safer sex. He doesn't understand the big deal about men who are on the DL. He said his wife doesn't ask him about such things because they have a relationship that is based on providing a good home for their children and being there for each other. He thinks that men who don't practice safer sex are the ones who make it bad for all the men who are not putting their sexual partners at risk. He supports the message of safer sex, but not the movement for men to come out and tell their women if they are on the DL.

The bottom line for him is that he feels that what he does is his business and he doesn't have to get permission to have sex on the DL. He doesn't feel compelled to have sex with men; he does it because he enjoys it. He told me that he is in touch with his sexual desires and he will pursue them. And all of this sounds perfectly fine until you realize that he's got a wife—maybe kids—at home who may one day find out about this other part of his life and be devastated by it.

One irony of DL behavior is that it sometimes cuts two ways: The DL brother can sometimes be simultaneously cheating on both ends of his life. The spouse or girlfriend at home may be a victim of his cheating ways, but the boyfriend or lover on the other end may also be surprised to discover that he's not in an exclusive relationship. This is how infidelity can work in our minds—the dishonesty isn't contained, it takes over everything. And the sting of infidelity has the same impact on everyone, no matter if you are in a homosexual relationship or a heterosexual relationship. I received an e-mail from a young man living in Baltimore, Maryland, recently who told me that he'd fallen in love with a man but later discovered that this man was having DL relationships all over the city. He shared this story with me.

I met a brother about four months ago and fell in love. He told me that he was a homebody and didn't do much socially but go to church, work, and hang out at home. We spent a lot of time together, and he was very attentive to me. I used to tell him that he was giving me too much of his time, and he told me that he wanted to spend all of his free time with me.

It wasn't long before I found out that he has three different lovers, men and women, scattered all over the city. Now I regret meeting him and allowing myself to get caught up in this screwed-up situation. I thought I knew what I was doing, but I guess now I didn't. I don't want to become a potential HIV/ AIDS victim from dealing with him, just because he doesn't know how to be a man and put all his cards on the table without lying. I don't want to have to pay for his lying, cheating, sneaky ways. In the long run he says he loves me, but that is clearly not true, because I don't think he even loves himself.

I am hurting. So, JL, please make it clear to the people you meet and speak to that DL behavior has the same impact on gay men, just like it does on women. Why can't people just be real and not drag others into their mess? All I wanted to do was to be in love with someone who wanted to be in love with just me.

—No Longer in Love

This was an interesting e-mail for me, because it shows that some DL men are not just in it for a quick hit of sex. The man who had seduced "No Longer in Love" did so by displaying signs of true love and commitment, not just a promise of a sexual thrill. This is why "No Longer in Love" felt genuinely betrayed.

This was something I began to discover as I listened to more and more stories of DL men. Some of them were out there looking for more than just sex, which was a revelation to me. I used to feel that DL men would never accept being with a man in a long-term relationship that was about more than just sex. In past presentations, I would tell my audiences that DL men would always have a woman in their lives, that they would never choose a man over a women, at least when it came to settling down in a long-term relationship. This was based on the evidence of the many men I'd met up to that point and on the evidence of my own thinking—at least as I thought at that time. I now stand corrected.

I've seen it in the men I've met, and I've seen it in my own life. I have now met and heard from many more brothers who were formerly on the DL. Many are a bit older, fathers who like me once lived a double life but now accept who they are and have chosen to be with a man. A lot of these men have informed their exwives and children, and now, in many cases, everybody is getting along just fine. It took some of the women awhile to accept it, but once they recovered, their relationships were healthier and more honest and, therefore, better for the children involved.

Then there are the former DL men who have told me that they still have to hide their SGL lifestyles because their families, professional colleagues, and friends would not accept them being with a man. They continue living their lives "in the closet," but with the big—and healthy—difference being that they've ceased to use women as fronts or sex objects. They've made a choice.

This is part of the change that is happening in the black community—a shift toward honesty. It's thrilling, even though it's still happening too slowly. As I said before, there has to be more acceptance in society before more men will feel able to expose their secret DL lives. Without the support and understanding of the community, these men will continue to deceive out of their own fear and confusion.

Being bisexual means that I have a choice when it comes to sexual partners, but the fact that I am a bisexual man does not mean that I will forever have multiple partners. I am often asked "Will you ever settle down with a man or a woman?" In the past–before I came around to admitting to my own bisexuality–I would have answered, "a woman" . . . and I would've given that answer in a hurry before anyone had time even to think about the other option! I was still operating with the residue of my old DL thinking, trying to put up a front to appear as close to "straight" as possible to avoid all of the consequences of truly coming out. But when I'm asked that question these days, my answer has changed. Now I feel free admitting the truth: I absolutely think I could develop a relationship with a man.

For me, in the end, it would have to come down to the qualities of the person, rather than their sex. I feel there comes a point in your life when you take a look at where you are and you decide what it would take to make you happy. Once you know what makes you happy, then you can find it. But, it takes honesty on your part.

Of course, I realize now that my life would've been much better if I'd explored all of this much earlier. But it was hard when I was younger. I didn't understand what I was. Was I a queer, gay, a faggot? I felt unaccepted in church, by my God. I couldn't make sense of it all. I ran every scenario through my head but just couldn't find one that would work for me. If I had the opportunity to openly explore my sexuality when I was younger, then maybe I would not have gotten married and been forced to put on the act that I did for so many years, just to please everybody else. I was afraid my church, friends, and family would find out about my bisexuality. And while I was having affairs with other men, thinking it was all top-secret, I suspected people were talking about me. Not talking, whispering. And when I was finally busted, I was still so scared to admit to what happened that I left the city. I hated the fact that I lost my marriage to my bisexuality, but at the same time, in retrospect, it was the best thing. I was glad, even then, that at least the lies were over and my secret was out and now both my life and the life of my exwife were free of that burden. I have always believed that everything happens for a reason, and looking back, I am glad that I got busted. I am glad that I was able to move on, and that my exwife was able to do so, too.

But I didn't immediately move on to an honest life. I was living on the DL for a very long time—before my marriage, during, and even when it ended. Way after the marriage was over, I was still in that DL mind-set. I was dating many beautiful women. I was a gentleman, well spoken, and many women were throwing themselves at me. One woman even bought me a brand-new SUV. I couldn't look her in the eye and tell her I loved her, because all I could think about was that I was fucking the guy next door. Despite all I'd learned about the importance of honesty from the fiasco of my own marriage's collapse, I still couldn't bring myself to be honest with the next women who came into my life.

Honesty is critical, as I said, but it can be so hard—particularly when in the grips of addiction. I know *addiction* is a strong word, but sexual addiction is real. And like any addiction, it short-circuits logic and rational thought. It makes you take stupid risks. When I was married—even when I had young children at home—I would take enormous risks to satisfy my seemingly unquenchable sexual appetite. I remember one particularly stupid incident vividly. I had some free time one day and spent it cruising this fine-looking man, tall and chiseled, at the ball courts, but we didn't hook up right then. Later that night, while I was lying in bed with my wife, I felt a tremor of intuition and decided to get up and take a look out of the window in my daughter's room, the window that faced the street outside of our home. There in the dim glow of the street lamps, I saw the man from the ball court outside my house, sitting in his car staring up at the window. Without thought, I motioned for him to come in. I creeped out of my daughter's room and down the stairs to the front door, careful not to wake anyone up. I unlatched the front door lock and there he was. Without a word he stumbled into the room and we fell on each other with an animal hunger and sexed each other down in front of the fireplace in my family's living room, just beneath my sleeping wife. When we were done, he hustled on out and I came back upstairs, hot from the sex and exhilarated by the thrill of getting away with such an outrageous act. It could only be the hold of a strong addiction that could explain such foolish, reckless behavior. It's my own experience that helps me understand stories like Lewis's.

Lewis is a twenty-nine-year-old married father of three who lives in a big city on the east coast. In his initial e-mail to me he stated:

Mr. King,

I just found out about your site. And I want to know if there is a cure for this type of behavior as I find it a hard cycle to break. Please help me. I am confused and need some help.

I wrote him back and we soon developed a regular correspondence via e-mail and over the phone. He shared with me that he was happily married and loved being a father but that he has struggled with his sexuality for all of his life. He was living on the down low and wanted to stop, but couldn't. He tried, but the desires kept coming back.

During one of our conversations, he was at home with the kids because his wife was getting her hair done. While we talked he was busy online cruising gay personal websites looking for men in his town to hook up with. I asked him if he was worried about his wife coming home, logging on, and checking out where he had been online. He said no, she isn't thinking like that. As far as he knew, she had no reasons to suspect him of looking at male-to-male personals. Theirs was a "normal" life, and he didn't feel he did anything to give her any hint about his double life. For her to even think he was on the DL was not a concern.

Then, sure enough, about a week later, he called to tell me that his wife had found some gay sites that he had been visiting. He was shocked that she found them, but I told him that when you get sloppy or overconfident, thinking that your woman isn't in touch with you and what you are doing, that's precisely when you get caught. Many men have gotten caught thinking their women are clueless.

Lewis pleaded with me to help him. He wanted to make a decision about how to go forward with his life. He was tired of lying and said he didn't have the strength to keep fighting what seemed like an uphill battle, a battle that he was losing.

I asked him what she said to him after she discovered he was surfing the net looking for men. He said that he lied to her and told her that a coworker had stopped by and used the computer one day when she was not at home. She said nothing else about it.

At the time they had been dealing with other issues in their marriage. They had been going to a marriage counselor for over a year, trying to work out some issues that had caused them to separate once. He had been cheating on his wife with a woman at his job; that woman had called his wife and told her about the relationship in hopes of breaking up his marriage so they could be together. His wife had been hurt, but she wanted to make their marriage work. She was willing to stick it out, and through counseling and prayer she felt that he would stop seeing other women, and he did. But he continued to see men on the side.

I understood where he was coming from. I understood the power of sexual hunger. But I told him that the bottom line is that he owes his wife the respect of giving her a choice. If she was willing to hang in there and help him work through his issues with his sexuality and apparent inability to control his sexual appetite, then wonderful. But if she wanted to leave him because of his trifling behavior, that was her choice, too. He was greedy for the control of the relationship—he wanted to have his cake and eat it, too. But if you truly love the person you're with, you have to look at the bigger picture and offer them a choice.

The other piece of advice I offer to people like Lewis is that if the need for sex overwhelms every other priority in their life, they should get professional help. Sexual addiction may seem funny—or even fun—but it's not. It's destructive. For me, I believe it started when I was a little boy—I would get my hands on any material that would stoke sexual desire. I would sneak glances at boys in the gym locker room changing clothes after dodgeball or glance over at men's penises when standing at a urinal. The more I saw, the more I wanted. I went further, grinding on a friend's leg when he fell asleep at a sleepover. I couldn't stop myself. Whatever shot I got to exercise my confusing sexual desires—whether for a man or a woman—I took, and it only made the feeling stronger. And as I grew older, and my sexual desires led me into a DL life, it never even felt like lying; it felt like fulfilling desire. I was just feeding the beast inside of me because I knew if I didn't, the desire would consume me. My behavior seemed perfectly justified; it was self-preservation.

That kind of need is a powerful thing. In all of our talk about honesty and fidelity and so on, we can't lose sight of that simple fact: Sex is perhaps the most powerful thing in the world. It's the drive that keeps the planet moving and the species alive. But we still have to control it. If that beast inside feels like it's lurching out of control, we have to remember to discipline desire—and to be aware of when we're losing our grip on it. And that's when you have to turn to someone you trust and talk it out. If you don't have access to professional help, then find anyone you trust—your pastor, a trusted friend, or a family member. Men in particular have tremendous difficulty talking freely about sex, unless they're bragging or telling tall tales. That was my problem, for sure.

When I went through my divorce, I realized that my sexual drive was out of control and causing me and my loved ones serious trouble. So I started to see a psychologist who specialized in working with young men. I went for six weeks, on Wednesday nights, and for the first three weeks I talked about everything under the sun except sex. But the psychologist just listened and read between the lines and created a nonjudgmental space that allowed me to talk around the subject until I was ready to address it head on. We didn't meet for very long, but he told me something that

I'll never forget: Until I learned to control my behavior, I'd always be in a vacuum of deception. In other words, out-of-control behavior actually *invites* deception. But the hopeful part of that message was the promise that if I dedicated myself to overcoming it, exercising will and discipline, it could be controlled. Sex is a powerful thing, but the human will can be even more powerful.

But that will goes both ways. Sometimes it's women who have to exercise will to end relationships that need to be ended and to look the truth in the eye. And even before the relationships take hold, it takes willpower to create safe, smart strategies for considering and entering intimate relationships.

When relationships are formed, there are so many emotions that play a part in that union, especially when sex is involved. If your partner is coming home later than usual, or checking his voicemail more often, curiosity will filter in. One woman e-mailed me that she feels that women take longer to process and digest emotional information than men. She thinks this is the reason women are quicker to settle for a man, any man, than wait for the right one. I am not sure if that is a true statement, but I do know that there is not enough planning or communication between couples before they become intimate.

My message to single sisters everywhere is to analyze your dating strategies. Protect your body and your heart. Do not assume, ask questions, and offer information. Make sure you have covered all bases before you decide to be intimate.

And if a brother reveals himself to be untrustworthy or duplicitous, and shows no signs of remorse or repentance, then it's important for you to act in your best interests. One sister told me that there is a thin line between love and hate and that she could stop loving her man in an instant if he wasn't honest with her. She said she would expect him to give her a choice and not place her in a situation that could hurt her. And she was willing to deal with that. She said if she was with a man who told her from day one that he was gay or bisexual, then it would be her choice if she wanted to be with him. But she didn't want to find out after the fact, after she had given him her body and love and had her emotions wrapped up, all in a lie.

I remember when I was dating a sister in D.C. many years ago. This sister really loved me. She was a single mother of three young daughters. She had not been involved with a man for several years prior to meeting me. When we met, she fell in love with me fast and hard. We had a good time together. She had a very strong sex drive, and she was one of those women who felt that the man comes first, and women were created to take care of their men. She would take care of me and even took a second job to support me when I was out of work. She didn't require a thing from me except for me to love her and be home with her at night.

Because I was not working, I had a lot of time on my hands. I would hang out at the mall or just ride around all day looking for something, anything to get involved with. During this time, I would meet other men who, like me, were not doing anything all day, just hanging out looking for something to get into. And sometimes that "thing" would be sex. I would pick up both men and women and get my freak on. I was bored, and since I had a high sex drive, I took this time to take care of my needs.

But every day at 5 p.m., I would be home waiting on my lady to come back. One weekend, she wanted me to attend a church affair with her and her sister, but I didn't want to go. I had made plans to hang out with one of my boys. She was not feeling that. When she laid out my clothes to wear that night, I told her that I was not going and left the house while she was in the shower. When I got home later that night, my key would not fit in the door, and there was a box sitting in the driveway. The box had all of my things in it. Everything. I knocked on the door and rang the doorbell, but she did not answer. I jumped in the car and left. I drove to a friend's house and started calling her, but she didn't answer the phone. The next morning, I got up early and went back to the house and parked my car outside on the curb. When she came out, I jumped out of the car and started a huge argument with her. I asked, "Why you tripping, putting my stuff out in the street . . . what's your problem?" She just walked past me, got in her car, and pulled away. I never heard from her again. She acted as if I didn't exist and she cut me off just like that. That situation taught me not to mess with a woman's feelings. Even though she didn't know that I was on the DL, she didn't want a man in her life that would not bend a little for her, especially if she was doing more for me than I was doing even for myself.

One day many years later, she told me that because I didn't attend that event with her, she could not continue the relationship. She said she knew that I was messing around on her, but she didn't care, because she was happy to have me in her life. And the other women might be getting the dick, but she had the total package. But when I had told her I would not attend the event, she had felt that I was going to go to *another* woman's house, and for that I had to go and be gone from her home and life. She and I never spoke about it again, and I can only assume she now knows my messing around was very likely with a man.

Every woman knows where her line is drawn, just like that sister did. And when that line gets crossed, you really have no choice but to act and act decisively in your best interests.

I'm going to end this discussion with the story of a DL man who is working hard to come up. It's men like this who inspire me and affirm to me that the most important thing for all of us—men, women, straight, gay, whatever—is to demonstrate true love in our dealings with one another and with ourselves. Love makes even the trickiest conversations possible—if not easy—and can help us find our way out of the most hopeless-seeming situations. Here's his story.

> I was getting tired of trying to live two lives. It was taking its toll on me and my family. My wife was beginning to ask me questions

about my love, our marriage, what was wrong with me. I was losing sleep at night and always wondering if I was HIV positive. And I was out of control, and no matter how I tried to control my desires, I always lost the internal battle. Then it finally happened. I got busted because I thought I was unstoppable. What happened is this:

I have a friend—I will call him Jesse. He lives in Virginia and is a minister with a moderate-size congregation. He was married and in a long-term relationship with another married minister. Jesse also slept with other men he met in various places, including the Internet. He was going through a very nasty divorce when I met him. We eventually became very close and became each other's lifeline of sorts. Jesse thought he had lost everything when he discovered that he was HIV positive. Everything he had worked for was slipping away, and there is the very real possibility that he had infected his wife and his friend. He was suicidal. I supported Jesse as best as I could.

On Christmas morning, I called Jesse to wish him Merry Christmas and Happy New Year, and to lend him continued support during his ordeal. The conversation became more involved than he planned. We started talking about the last man we had been with, and how good the sex was. I was telling him about this dude I met online and how we had sex at a local motel and we were scheduled to hook up again in a couple of days. When the called ended, I looked up and my wife was standing there. She had heard the entire conversation. I was in shock and knew that I had to come clean and admit that I was bisexual. My wife and I had an intense discussion, and we even considered the possibility of divorce. She said the trust she thought we had been working to rebuild was gone and she could no longer be in a relationship where she felt she was being played. We agreed to call a therapist for an emergency session to find out what to do next. Later that day, I called a close friend who I had been involved with over the past two years—a really nice gay man who taught me the ropes of being with men, and a brother who I had learned to trust and lean on when I was meeting different men. He was the man in my life who educated me about HIV and the risk that I was putting myself and my wife in. This brother was someone who I fell in love with. I had to call him and tell him that we might have to end our friendship, this time for good. I had tried in the past to end my relationship with him, but I couldn't stay away. The sex we had was awesome and I loved him as a person. I called him and then before he could say anything I ended the phone call.

After Christmas passed, I called him as I waited for an HIV clinic to open. I told him how my wife and I had sat with the therapist and really opened up for the first time. I told him that after therapy, we sat in the car for several hours, just talking and crying together. The strength of the communication continued as we got home. Eventually, we made passionate love. It had been several months since we last had sex. It was the closest that I had felt to my wife in years. Then she told me that she was pregnant. At that point, I decided to be completely forthright with my wife and told her everything—that I had an ongoing relationship with a man. She was stunned, but expressed that she thought all of this was happening to her because she had an abortion at nineteen. We felt that we needed to consider everything for the sake of the kids. We decided we would continue with the therapy to determine if my need to be with men was a result of some sexual addiction or if I was inherently bisexual, where no amount of therapy could change anything. She made it clear that she did not want to share her husband emotionally with anyone else. If I wanted to remain married to her, I had to break all ties with my friend and any other men she viewed as a threat to our marriage. If I found that I had a true emotional need to be with another man, we would divorce and it would be unlikely for her to remarry.

With divorce as an option, scenarios were discussed with regard to the kids, including living under the same roof in different rooms with different lives or maintaining separate residences. She said she would have no problem with me having other people around the kids. We could sell the house and she would move to another city with shared custody of the kids. I didn't want to lose my children and was adamant that I remain in the lives of my kids at all costs, because I had been deprived of my father when my parents divorced. My parents had gone through a bitter divorce and I felt forced to choose between my mother and father. I didn't want my kids to experience any of that. My wife and I both agreed that if we got a divorce, it would not be messy, and no one would win.

Perhaps the biggest news was that if it was determined through therapy that I was inherently bisexual and I felt I couldn't contain my desires to be with men, I would come out to my family. I figured that if I could share my greatest struggle so openly with the most important person in my life, I could be just as honest with my mother, father, and brother.

Twenty minutes after I got my HIV test results, I called my lover to tell him that I was negative. I told him I loved him and he would always be in my heart, but I had to move on and try to save my marriage. I told him that my wife and my family meant more than life to me and I was going to work on healing all the hurt that I put on my family. And the only way I could do that was to cut all ties to anyone that was a part of my life on the DL. Then I said good-bye.

When I got home I took my laptop and totally cleaned out all the personal gay websites that I had put in a file. I deleted every phone number in my cell of men I had met and who had become part of my "stable," and I started opening up with my wife. We are growing closer and closer every day. It feels good to talk to her about my feelings, struggles, and even my desires for sex with men. She has not judged me, but tells me that together we will get through this and we will keep God first in our life.

3

THERE ARE NO SIGNS

Ladies, you sure are persistent. Even after *Oprah*, my first book, the countless speaking engagements, my website, and the radio and magazine interviews, you are still asking me that million-dollar question: *What are the signs?* You still want to know what to look for and how you will be able to tell if your man is on the down low.

I have told women across the country that there are no signs, and their only defense is their intuition. And if they are feeling that something is *not right* with their mate, then chances are they're right. That little voice inside speaking to them is talking for a reason. If they're hearing from that little voice, then it's time to get nosey. Ask questions, but in a loving, nonconfrontational way. The goal is to get the behavior out in the open, or to get yourself reassured. But trying to play like Nancy Drew and the Hardy Boys—or like some kind of FBI profiler—is not going to help. Keeping tuned to your intuition and creating an open environment that allows for free sexual discussion is really the best solution.

But it doesn't matter what I say: Women want me to show them the "look" or to tell them if I can spot any DL men in the room. And if there is a DL man in the room, they want me to spot him and give him the look, so they can see how a DL hookup happens. Many of the women who show up to my presentations attend with this one mission in mind: to find out what the foolproof signs are. Many have gotten upset with me when I don't give them a detailed answer or tell them what they want to hear.

I beg women to stop the accusations and to stop looking for signs. The truth is there really are no concrete signs. DL men do not have a secret handshake or special wink. They do not have a membership card or code word. It is not that deep. DL men often find each other in the crowd through the kind of communication that happens subtly and unconsciously, not through some kind of explicit hand signal. When you know what you're looking for, you know when you've found it.

I feel like all this attention placed on *the signs* is a way for some women to disconnect themselves from their instinctive and intuitive feelings. Many feel that if their man isn't sending them *the signs,* then whatever made them question their man's sexuality in the first place is null and void. This may be wishful thinking.

On the other hand, please remember that not all men practice this lifestyle. So do not put every man you come into contact under the microscope. And please do not obsess over this; you have to leave room in your life to live and love. Not all men are sneaking around having sex with other men. I'll admit that in my first book I tried to be as clear as possible about the threat of DL men, but only because I know that threat is real and can be deadly. But I do not suggest that every woman on the planet has to live in constant fear of the DL lifestyle.

I do, however, suggest that couples in relationships start communicating with each other. Sex, as one of the components of a mature adult relationship, should be a subject that is always open for conversation. If you are adult enough to engage in sex, you should be adult enough to communicate about it with the person you are doing it with. If you're really getting to know a person, you should ask candid questions, listen to your heart, and follow that "little voice" that tells you what's right and wrong. I've talked to woman after woman about this in my travels, and the bottom line is that looking for signs can be an empty exercise, but creating an environment for open communication about sex is never a wasted effort.

Still, in order for me to settle the minds of those who need to know what the signs are, I share with them a story of a sister from D.C. who asked me to find out if her man was on the DL. For reasons she couldn't quite put her finger on, she had a feeling that something wasn't right. Though the thought had crossed her mind on many occasions to confront him about it, she never did. She told me that she loved him and even if something wasn't right, she would try to work the relationship out. She wanted him to be happy, but even more so, she wanted him to be honest with her. So we set him up.

She and I planned that I would bump into them at a restaurant. We would act like old friends and she would introduce me to him. Once I was at their table and talking to her about old times, she would excuse herself from the table, leaving him and me to get to know each other better. We set the plan into action. Once the two of us were alone, I suggested to him that since I only had one night in town that later in the evening the two of us should get together so he could take me to some clubs for fun. I even suggested that we go to a strip club to check out the ladies. He was cool with the idea.

Later that evening he met me at my hotel. He called me from the lobby and I told him I was still getting dressed, so he should just come up. I opened the door in my towel and told him to come in and have a drink while I got ready. We talked about sisters in town and I even mentioned that tonight I was feeling extra horny. As I was getting dressed I noticed him staring at me. I stopped buttoning my shirt and looked him right in his eyes. The contact was long enough to let me know that he was interested. I asked him if going out was not what he really had in mind, "or would you rather just get with me." He said yes and soon we started kissing and rubbing. We finally made our way over to the bed. I had no intentions of having sex with him; I was not attracted to him like that, not to mention the fact that he was already in a relationship with a woman I was trying help. He, on the other hand was asking me to take him and do what I wanted with him. We had already established what we both liked to do sexually: He was a bottom and I'm a top. While we kissed and rubbed he actually moaned out that he wanted me to penetrate him right there. There were no condoms mentioned by either of us. Sometimes in cases of quick hook-ups like this, the man getting penetrated will trust that the top is going to use a condom or he'll simply hope the top doesn't have any STDs. A lot of bottoms leave it up to the top to make this important decision. Sometimes if there has been drinking or drug use, or the sex is for money, or lust has completely taken over all common sense, condoms will be the furthest thing from the minds of either party.

Anyway, at this point I got up and went to the bathroom, locked the door, and called out that I wasn't feeling well. I yelled through the door that I had a sharp pain in my stomach. He ended up sleeping in the room with me that night without any more intimacy and then going back home in the morning. When his girl called me the next day, I told her what happened. After digesting this information, she decided that before confronting him, she would first give him a chance to be honest with her.

She asked him several times during a period of three days if he had ever been curious or thought about having sex with a man. He said no. She asked him if he had ever been approached by a man for sex. Again he told her no. He said that he hated gay men, and if one ever approached him he would probably end up in jail, because he would hurt that person. After three days of lying to her, she had to make a decision based on the proof that I had given her. She was hurt and scared but knew that she had to make a choice about her future. She decided to end her engagement to him. She then took an HIV test, which sadly came back positive. When she called him to confront him and tell him about her test results, he hung up on her and moved out of town. Since that day, she has not heard from him.

I remember when she first called me to ask if I would do her this favor and check him out. I told her that if she had to ask, then she already knew something was not right. I remember telling her that she didn't need me to check him out; all she had to do was follow her "inner voice" and, of course, ask him. I suggested she at least try to get him to listen and talk about what she was feeling. I also told her that I hoped she was ready for what the results would be from my findings. I wanted to prepare her for the bad news and I also wanted her to realize that she didn't need me to justify what she already knew deep inside.

I have gay friends who tell me that some female friends ask them to turn on their "gaydar" and let them know what's up with the new man in their lives. Many of them have busted these guys, and the female friends are usually shocked when they find out. One gay man told me that he took his best female friend to a gay club and showed her the man she was in love with dancing with another brother. And another gay friend of mine always jokes that if a girl really needs to know about her man she should just call him. He was thinking about opening up a private detective agency to bust DL men. He told me that he could make millions of dollars. Plus, he told me that finding out if a man was on the DL is the easiest thing in the world, like taking candy from a baby, and he was up for the challenge. When I ask sisters if they would pay for that type of service, all of them say, *"Hell yeah."* So, I guess my friend is on to something.

But questions about the signs keep coming. Here are some examples:

> Hello JL,
>
> First of all, I want to thank you for your information on living on the down low. I have a girlfriend who is seeing this guy, Tom, who has a gay male friend. She is very uncomfortable with their "friendship."
>
> Well, one morning around 7 a.m., my girlfriend called Tom, and his gay friend answered the phone. He got upset with my girlfriend and told her that Tom was sleeping!
>
> You'd think bells would go off in my girlfriend's head. But it's like she still doesn't want to break it off completely with Tom. She says she needs to know for sure . . . and that she is going to ask Tom in a roundabout way whether he is gay or not. I'm like helllllooooooo! Just the suspicion of a guy being gay will make me run the other way!
>
> Is it normal for a straight black male to have a platonic relationship with an openly gay male? How can I help my girlfriend?
>
> Thanks for any help!

This is one of the so-called signs that I come across all the time. There are a lot of women who get nervous if their man has a lot of gay friends, particularly if any of them are close friends. And, yes, it's not the norm for straight men to hang around a set of gay men. But we have to allow for the full range of acceptable social behavior before we let our imaginations run away with us. Whether or not this woman's boyfriend is gay or not is certainly not clear from this short e-mail, but there really shouldn't be a problem with him being friends with a gay man. But if this sister's intuition is humming, she should still ask some questions.

> Hi,
>
> I just want your opinion. When I was dating this guy, the very first time we had sex, he kept guiding my finger toward his rectum. I thought that odd for a heterosexual guy. But in any event, it turned me off, and I stopped seeing him after that. Do you think he was a DL brother?

Sometimes we get caught up by our own lack of sexual experience. Sex is a crazy thing. There's almost no limit to what turns people on or what they do when the lights are low and the door's locked. There are many straight men—not to mention women—who love anal stimulation of various kinds during sex. So, no, a desire to get your booty smacked up, flipped, or rubbed down (or even more) is not necessarily relevant to your sexual orientation.

> Dear JL,
>
> Can you let me know what you think about a man that urinates with the seat down like a woman? Is this a sign? This man

is very masculine, but he likes to take bubble baths and buy bubble bath from the Bath & Body Works store. He says that he is buying this for himself!

He loves nice, expensive candles all over the entire house. He is forty-two, handsome, and has a professional job. Never been married and says that he is not ready for a commitment or is scared of commitment. Last question, what if he keeps testing me by asking me if I want to try sex in the anus? I keep saying no and ask him why. He would say he is curious. He thinks that I am just kidding by telling him I do not want sex in the anus and that it is SODOMY according to the Bible and there are consequences.

Please let me know what you think about the questions I have asked you. Thank You.

Okay, as for how the man urinates—I can't explain it. Maybe he's tired! Gay men urinate standing up for the most part, just like other men. It doesn't mean anything. And men are allowed to pamper themselves, too, without having their sexuality called into question. Finally, anal sex with women is a turn-on for many straight men; again, it's not relevant to their sexual orientation.

Dear JL,

I'm a black thirty-five-year-old woman. I've known my husband for a total of six and a half years. Two years before we decided to move in together, he was living with his father.

One particular day I was on his computer about to use the Internet and I scrolled down to find aol, because I was about to check my e-mail. What I also saw was a shemale website. I immediately started breathing heavy, almost about to pass out. Just to take you back for a minute, there've been plenty of times I've spent the night at his house and he didn't touch me once. A lot of times I tried to blame it on school, because at the time he was attending a technical/vocational college and didn't get in until late, so I just figured he was tired. We had sex every Sunday afternoon. It became so predictable and boring. Back then he was a private kinda guy, and mostly I think it was because his dad would be in the house and he was afraid that I would be moaning loud. But it just would not sit well with me, because what was always running through my mind was "if I was in any other man's bed he would not refuse me or make me wait for sex," not that I think I'm all that or anything, but I'm attractive in many ways and I can't deny that.

O.K.

Fast-forward back to the Internet situation. I asked him, "What is this?" and he quickly got angry and replied, "It's not mine, I don't know. It's probably my uncle's." (But his uncle did not spend as much time on that computer as he did, and was barely even home.) I said to my love, if you were not looking this up on the Internet you wouldn't be getting so upset about it (I mean, he was about to damn near cry). So I left as fast as I could to get myself together, came back, and he was still explaining, "Why would you think it was mine?"

When we moved in together (not married yet), I was looking in his e-mail inbox because I had put his résumé on several job sites and I was trying to see if anyone responded to them. I found letters with the subjects shemale this and shemale that. I confronted him and said, "What's up with this, because now you can't blame it on your uncle," and he said when he goes on other sites like bigblackbooty.com, nudeafrica.com, etc., they send it automatically as junk mail.

Once we were living together we did have more sex, and when we got married he really came out of his shell. A few weeks after we married, we visited some of his family members in the North. He really surprised me up there. I thought we would never have sex up there because he's such a private guy and we were staying with different family members. I said to him, "I'm shocked you're gonna really give me some with your dad and family in the house." He responded, "I don't care, girl. You're my wife I can do what I want with my wife."

—Help Me to Understand

P. S. I've even asked him if he's ever wanted to sleep with a man and of course he said NO.

Sexual fantasy is a completely unpredictable thing. There are lots of people—maybe all of us—who are turned on by things that we also think are perverse. Again, while this correspondent is right to question what's up when she finds "shemale" porn, the surprising answer might be that it's just something that turns him on as a fantasy, but not something he ever wants to pursue in his actual life.

Hey JL,

On the subject of "down low," I was dating this guy that I suspected of being a "down low" brother even though he had two baby mommas. I tried to justify the types of friends he had because of his line of work (he works in a night club), but some of the things he did and didn't do in bed, and the increasing number of his friends who "looked" gay, worried me to the point that I called it off. He is unaware of why I called it off because I don't know how to confront him about my fears. Should I just continue to go on ignoring him and his phone calls or say something?

This really is the problem with looking for signs. It can hurt you in two ways: If your man fails to exhibit what you think the signs are, you relax your guard, not realizing that just because he puts on a good act doesn't mean he's not creeping out on you. On the other hand, if we make decisions based on these so-called signs, instead of based on open and honest communication, we can end up wrongfully accusing a perfectly innocent person and destroying a worthwhile relationship.

On your website you have a link called "Why I Do What I Do." It explains why you came out about your life on the down low. But that doesn't explain to me why you do what you do in the sense of why you chose to be a down-low brotha. Where is the explanation for that? I am a sista and very weary about this whole down-low-brotha situation. If we are supposed to understand the situation, then how can we understand if we don't know why brothas do it. Also, if these brothas are on the down low and going to lie about it anyway, how are sistas going to be able to protect ourselves. What are the signs?

I feel where this sister is coming from. I know it's wearying and confusing and I know that most of all, you

want to know if there are signs. But the problem is that
brothers are on the down low for many different reasons
and they do their dirt in many different ways; the most
important thing I tell women I meet is not to worry about all
the down-low brothers in the world, but to focus on the
man in front of them. Just as in all other facets of life, you
need to look for a man who can be open and honest about
his sex life and who's willing to do the work of making you
feel secure.

When women tell me that they're looking for signs, what
they usually mean is they're looking for what they think are
obvious behavioral signs, like the ones associated with a
stereotypical gay man. But my own case is proof that that's
not necessarily going to work. My wife never questioned me
about my sexuality until she had proof, and none of my
women ever asked me about my sexuality. Even my friends
never once questioned me about my sexuality. I never
exhibited those traits. Even today, as a confident bisexual
man, I do not wear my sexuality on my sleeve. And back
when I was DL, I wasn't conducting myself like a stereotypical gay man. I wasn't flamboyant or feminine. I remember
hanging out with coworkers or close male friends and laughing at gay jokes. I would even turn around and tell a good
joke myself, as ridiculous as that was. Gay was just not something I associated myself with. I never thought that what I
was doing was gay. I just thought I was a freak and that getting my penis sucked by a man was just that . . . getting my

dick sucked. So the fact is that just because a man comes across as hard or manly or even homophobic, there's no guarantee that he's not on the DL.

And the opposite is true, too. If a man comes across soft or fem, it does not make him gay. I have many friends who are small in body stature and who in their style and body language act like stereotypical gay men, but these men are 100 percent heterosexual. They get upset when people joke about them because they don't like sports, but the truth is they prefer shopping and pampering themselves. And, I repeat, they're 100 percent heterosexual. I know many straight men who love going to the theater, or who cry at emotional movies, but they feel almost as if they have to apologize for having these traits. I have a very close friend who wants to take a dance class but is afraid that people will think he is gay.

This sort of thing is ridiculous. Any man who is coming across as overtly, dramatically, visibly gay probably is and, more important, will tell you if asked. A demonstrably gay man is not trying to hide his sexuality. He probably has no interest in being confused for straight, and will set *you* straight on that if he has to. Many out and proud SGL men and women don't hide their sexual orientation and take offense at those who do.

On the other hand, no man or woman on the DL is going to give signs. That would defeat the purpose of being on the *low*. Their greatest fear is giving off overt signs and signals that will get them busted; they don't even want there to be the smallest hint of public confusion about their sexuality because at heart they are ashamed and scared of their own confusion. Their MO is deceit, and once you're practiced in the arts of deception, you learn not to blow it with silly, easy-to-spot signals. The practiced liar is way too slick for that. When you're on the DL, the lies you devise to cover your tracks can be as simple as arithmetic or as complicated as calculus.

I remember when I was dating this fine, smart, ambitious sister who had a high-power, high-profile position. She came home early one day to find me in bed with a brother who I had met at the mall. When she walked into the bedroom we were asleep, and I didn't wake up till I heard the bedroom door slam. I rolled out of bed without really thinking and got up to check on the noise. When I stepped into the hallway I saw my girl sitting at the kitchen table drinking a Coke, looking agitated. I was standing there naked and momentarily shocked. But I wasn't new to this. I didn't panic. I knew I had to regroup and regroup fast. If I overreacted then it would just make it look like I was guilty of something, so I played it cool. I just walked over to her, kissed her on the forehead, and went back into the bedroom and shut the door. She left the house a little while after that. When she came home later, she didn't say anything and neither did I. I was not going to mention it, and my strategy was simply to act as if nothing happened. In my mind I was thinking that if *she* brought it up, I would make sure that whatever she thought she saw, I'd spin it and flip it until she started to question her own eyes and memory.

There Are No Signs

On the way to a dinner party that night, she finally brought it up. I told her that I met this brother at the mall who gives massages in the nude. I said that I'd invited him to the house to massage me and it was so good that I fell asleep, and when I woke up he was lying beside me asleep, too. When she looked skeptical, I explained to her that the massages are done in the nude to ensure a better exchange of energy. I threw in that we drank a bottle of wine before the massage. She knew that I enjoyed a nice glass of wine before I got a massage. My mind was racing, but on the surface I was cool. I played it off like it was no big deal, no drama, and when I was done, I made it clear that I was not going to explain anything further. And she never asked another question. When we got home that night, I made sure I rocked her world, and trust me, if she had any suspicion about whether or not I was straight, that session made her forget.

This is the classic way a down-low brother can get over on a woman who spends all her time looking for signs. Because I kept up the appearance of a very masculine man and put it down on her in the bedroom, she kept quiet about her concerns. But at the same time, she ignored the evidence that was right in front of her eyes. She caught me in bed, naked, with another man. But she still let me slide with some fast-talking lies and an outward display of masculinity.

This is how some men get over. Some DL men are downright scornful of women—they say that "women will accept anything," and sometimes, sad to say, they're right. This particular woman was dealing with a familiar set of circumstances. She was smart, lovely, and successful, but lonely. She hadn't had a man in her life for a long time before she met me. She'd watched a succession of her friends get married and felt trapped in the "always a bridesmaid" cliché. When we hooked up, it was both exciting for her and a relief. Finally, she had a tall, dark, church-going brother to take around town, a man who'd lavish her with attention. I won her trust and love—and I had her where I wanted her. At that point, since I knew I hadn't given her any obvious signs that would make her uncomfortable or embarrass her in front of her friends and family, I knew I was home free— to the point where I could get caught in the act and still not have her turn me out.

So what's the lesson of this story? To any person desperately searching for signs, stop. Women, please stop spending your time and energy looking for signs. Again, it is not about *signs*, it is about facts. Actual facts that prove your man is on the DL. If he's on the DL, he'll give you no signs because he doesn't want to get caught. If he was comfortable and secure in his sexuality he would have told you about it by now. He's not, which is why he's hiding it for all he's worth. In the DL community there are only signs to connect one brother to another, not signs thrown out to the rest of the world just to get caught. The dilemma of looking for signs is that by searching too hard and interrogating loved ones, you'll end up ruining good relationships. And by focusing on superficial behavior and ignoring *true* evidence, you can end up sustaining a relationship that perhaps should end.

Not everyone subscribes to my "no signs" theory. Some feel that there has to be something besides basic human intuition. One physician, Beverly Coleman-Miller, debated this with me at the "Black Love II: Dating, Disease, and the Down Low" during the 34th Congressional Black Caucus Legislative Conference in Washington, D.C. She stepped up to the microphone as the people were filing out and loudly and passionately spoke about her theory, which is that, as a medical professional, she's seen *physical* signs that prove or at least strongly suggest that someone is on the DL. Although when I say there are no signs, I'm speaking primarily about behavioral signs, not physical signs, I'm skeptical of Dr. Coleman-Miller's theories about physical signs. But in fairness, I'm going to let her explain her position:

The beautiful young black women and handsome young men standing in line outside the closed doors of the conference room manifested their curiosity and uncertainty about this down-low issue. They were polite to one another but mostly focused on the possibility that the doors might open and the security guard would allow them into the standing-room-only, can't-violate-the-fire-department rules panel presentations in which Mr. J. L. King was a participant. As a physician involved in reducing AIDS through education, I needed to hear the presentations. The content of the last question in the session was the one that everyone was most curious about: "Mr. King, how do you know when a man is on the down low?" Mr. King slowly moved the microphone toward him and tapped it to make sure it was working. Then, he leaned forward, looked directly into the crowd of the curious, and said in a clear, deep voice, *"Intuition."*

Mr. King is probably correct. His book describes intuition as the best detector. I wanted that to be an acceptable answer for this complex question. But then there is the problem that 73 percent of newly diagnosed HIV/AIDS patients are black women. I knew those women needed an answer that would reduce some of their helplessness and allow them to walk out of that room wrapping their minds around the reality of the down low just as their man wraps his arms around them. As I stood to speak, they knew intuition was killing them. Anything I said would help. When I started to speak, they cheered and encouraged me to continue.

Words like *saliva, ejaculate,* and *anus* came out of my mouth in a series of run-on sentences about sex acts. Quiet prevailed in the room, dotted with an occasional amen. I reminded them that as a nurse and a doctor I have seen the anus (area of insertion of the penis when men have sex with men) of the young, the constipated, the incontinent, the old, the gay, the raped, the heterosexual-female-who-does-anal-sex, the transvestite, and more. In our professions, we have done prostate exams, diagnosed hemorrhoids, delivered babies, and we have seen all kinds of infections "down there." We have swabbed anuses and we have asked the surgeons to sew up some after a violent act. Anuses and behaviors around that area of the body have been a part of every health professional's life. We know a lot about the physical consequences of sex and J. L. King has brought the subject to the table for discussion.

Mouths have also been part of our lives. Our patients allow a tongue depressor to be placed on their tongues so that the tonsils can be examined. We have seen some almost vomit when the tongue is extruded and we have seen some allow the tongue depressor halfway down their throat with no problem. We know some who did not need the depressor for their tonsils to be visible.

None of this necessarily proves anything. None of it confirms that any man is on the down low. There are limitations to the idea of physical indicators. There are more limitations to intuition. If intuition works, it can reduce AIDS exponentially. Along with intuition, however, it may be advisable to translate basic knowledge into something that will lead to even more questions that may, in turn, lead to some consequential truths. From there, who can predict what can happen?

I have the utmost respect for medical doctors who work within the community and provide care to HIV-positive men and women. When Dr. Coleman-Miller and I agreed to work together to get a message out that would help, and we agreed that both of us could educate our community, I wanted her voice in this book. Because she feels strongly that there are physical signs, I felt that she needed to be heard. But there are some limitations to her suggestions about examining mouths and anuses for signs of DL behavior. For instance, not all gay men get anally penetrated, so what would be the physical signs for those men? The larger issue is that it would be very unusual for a man's wife or girlfriend to request or administer her own private anal exam or throat culture on her man. Can you imagine? Even now men and women are having it out over simple questions—imagine if women were trying to sneak in anal exams while their men slept? It would be disastrous and, ultimately, ineffective.

Accusation and interrogation are not the solutions. To the degree that there are signs that can be concealed, a man who is intent on staying on the DL will figure out how to conceal them. The only surefire solution is making sure there is sufficient caution before you enter into any intimate relationships, and that communication is open and honest from the beginning.

4

CHANGE IS POSSIBLE

I have met many DL men on both a personal and professional level. Prior to my first book, it was strictly because they were part of my secret world. As my life started changing and my secrets were exposed, I realized that my contact with these men was becoming more intense, ironically, as it became less sexual. I actually got to know these brothers on a different, more personal level. During my speaking engagements, the few men who showed up would listen intently while I told my story. Some were on the DL and some were not. I could tell by their eyes that they were searching for answers in my words. Many would arrive after the crowd had settled in and would sit in the back. And before the event was over, they would slip out the way they came in, quietly and unnoticed. The more engagements I did, the more cities I visited, the more DL men I would encounter. But not every man who came to these events would sneak out. I would speak with some men after the conferences and stay in touch with a few of them, some of whom have allowed me to interview them for this book.

Sometimes, while on tour, I'd encounter men who'd never been physically intimate with another man but wanted to. These men would sometimes approach me and subtly—or not so subtly in some cases—suggest that although they'd never been with a man, they were hoping I would be their first. At times I felt like these men were sitting around just waiting for me to run through their town so they could fulfill a desire they had long suppressed! But I know a lot of these men were just looking to reach out so they wouldn't feel so alone in their struggle, and like so many of us, they translated that reaching out into sex. There were other brothers who were already in the life, living DL, but they wanted me to know that I wasn't alone in the struggles I described.

But not all the feedback I've gotten from DL men has been positive. I've received hateful e-mails from angry black men pissed off because of my work and message. These are men who were upset because their women were now starting to ask them questions and watch them a bit closer. Some told me that they were upset because they overheard their wives talking to friends about my book or saw it covered on TV, and all this exposure was bringing the issue a little too close to home. They felt that what they did was their business and were alarmed at all the sudden attention on the subject. Others have boasted to me that no matter what I said, they weren't worried about being busted because their prowls were so calculated that their women would never suspect that they were on the DL.

I have been accused of inaccurately portraying African American men as the only group that is on the DL. Because of this, I have reworked my conferences. I am specific when I do interviews to not confuse the listener and have them think that only black men are on the DL. Likewise, I have taken steps to underscore that not all black men are on the DL. I even hang a sign on the stage as a backdrop with the message: NOT ALL AFRICAN AMERICAN MEN ARE ON THE DOWN LOW. I have the audience say it with me. I make it a point to acknowledge the men in the room and give them props for attending the event. I tell black women that they should not give up on finding a brother who will love them and not lie to them, and I make sure they understand that there are brothers out there who are not confused about their sexuality, men who won't lie to them about their sexual orientation. I have told my own daughter it's okay if she doesn't have a man, but I don't want her to give up on finding a black man because of my message. This is important to the future of the African American community. We need to promote marriages, commitment, and fidelity and make sure that our men are not feeling hunted or accused of being or doing something that they are not. My sons are not on the DL, and I don't want them to be accused of it because of me or simply because they are black.

But the feedback that gives me the most hope comes from those men who have shared with me that they have changed their behavior, put an end to their DL lives, and no longer deceive their loved ones—or themselves—about their sexual identity. These men are now clear about their sexuality and have nothing to hide anymore. Some of these men have chosen to be only with a man, and some are seeking counseling to deal with their sexual identity issues. I have heard many of these men tell me that while going through this process, they are living abstinent lives, so as not to complicate anyone else's life and put them at risk of great emotional pain—not to mention the potential health risks that come from unsafe promiscuity of any kind.

There are still many DL men out there that have sex with men, but many are careful to practice safer sex. One brother told me that the idea that all DL men don't protect themselves is an unfair and inaccurate judgment that has been placed on DL men. He himself claims that he is a man that always uses condoms and he is not out having carefree sex. He believes himself to be a responsible DL brother. And he's right: just because a brother is on the DL doesn't mean he's some kind of superpredator trying to spread HIV. In other words, just because a man is dishonest about his sexuality and unfaithful in his sexual affairs, it doesn't mean that he's necessarily also unsafe about his health and the health of his sexual partners. But it's not a huge leap from one kind of sexual irresponsibility to another—it's wise to stay away from sexual partners who exhibit irresponsibility of any kind.

I can only hope that as I continue to speak and spread my message that more men see the light and break free from this behavior. I know that my book and lectures have already had an impact on many lives. For the most part, the e-mails and letters I receive encourage me to keep speaking. The personal encounters with pained and confused men only convince me that my message must be heard. And the wonderful stories from the men that have changed breathes life into my journey.

In my first book I introduced five DL behavior types. I focused on their behavior based on their background, age, region, lifestyle, and education. These types were created based on my research, my 2,500 interviews, and my personal relationships. When I would meet a man that was over forty and he shared with me how he would do his DL thing, I would go back and read my notes of another brother who was over forty and compare their behavior. I was surprised at how many of the same behaviors fit those men, which became the basis for my profile of the Mature Brother. I would do this behavior/lifestyle comparison with every man that I interviewed. At the end of my research, I came up with several profiles, each profile a composite of many men who fit the category. This list is not based on any scientific theory, but rather the results are drawn from my anecdotal research.

In the past year I have had many DL men come up to me and say that a specific profile fit them perfectly, and seeing it on paper made them feel uneasy. They felt exposed after reading such a close account of their behavior and realized the pain they were causing. Many of these men have been compelled to change their DL behavior and have asked me to share their stories. Ironically, they admitted to me that if their daughter, niece, sister, mother, or female friend were involved with a DL man, they would be enraged and want to kill him if he hurt her.

I have continued conversations with them and have gotten a first-hand look into the lives of men who are coming up from the down low. These men were candid and honest with me, and that was the first step to *change*. Some have since admitted to themselves and their loved ones that they were selfish in their decisions. I have shared some very personal stories with these men, and they have returned the openness with me. The only request was that I not reveal their identity in the book. Some are still going through the first stages of admitting to their problem, while others are at a more advanced stage of healing. But the exciting thing about revisiting these types now is that each of them is trying to make a change.

In delivering my message of hope and the possibility of change, I want to be clear that my goal is not to present false hope. Some men, like myself, have changed and no longer live their lives on the down low. Others are contemplating their break from that lifestyle. And then there are others that will never change. The DL is not going to disappear because of my work. Nor will it come to a stand still when the media hype and buzz is gone. I wish it were that simple. I do not want to set any traps for women and I don't want to deliver a message that women should feel safe about practicing unprotected sex and not worry about men lying to them. Change is happening right now, but slowly, one life at a time. We have a long, long way to go before all DL men feel comfortable to come out in the open about their sexuality. Until we can start dealing with homophobia in every community—but the black community especially—some men will feel forced to stay in the closet and some of those will creep on the DL. This is a reality that I have lived.

Each of these profiles is unique in background, experience, and attitude toward sexuality. The stories here are real, although I've included details from various men to create a composite character in each case, in order to keep their identities concealed. Here are the types (readers of my first book will notice that the types are slightly revised from the five types I introduced in that book):

The Professional

The Guy Next Door

The Urban Brother

The Mature Brother

THE PROFESSIONAL

This man is typically a business professional or entrepreneur. He is college educated and financially secure. He often puts his work before his family or friends and has a bachelor mentality. Although he dates often, he has not been in a serious relationship in his adult life. He is trying to live the American Dream of life, liberty, and the avid pursuit of happiness.

I met professional brother Leroy, a thirty-six-year-old Atlanta corporate executive, at a cocktail party in Baltimore. He shared with me that one of his goals before he turned forty was to become a CEO of a Fortune 500 company, and because of his very demanding workload and the demands of keeping his "eye on the prize," he didn't have time for relationships. He dates women about three times a month, with almost all of those dates ending in one-night stands. In a very blunt and to-the-point manner, Leroy would lay out the rules to women who wanted to date him. Rule number one: no attachments. He is a no-nonsense kind of guy with a very specific agenda.

Leroy came to one of my lectures and afterward told me he wanted to talk to me. So we left the event and headed to a local Starbucks. I could tell by the look in his eyes that something was weighing heavily on his mind. He was excited about meeting me, and was not going to let me leave without sharing his story:

When I was thirty, I got married to get divorced. All the other fast-track guys were married with kids, making all of it happen.

But being a black man in corporate America, I knew I had to work harder. I didn't want the stress of a marriage, kids, and a demanding career, so I chose my work. The divorce was a sure thing because I wasn't there most of the time anyway. I was always away on business.

Funny thing is, during the last few months of our marriage, we started growing close to each other. For a few months, I even thought that we could make something work, but in the end, we wrapped things up and moved on. That made my life at work a lot easier because everyone knew I was divorced and I didn't have to deal with any suspicion about my life outside of work. They knew I was committed to career success.

Because of the traveling involved with my work, I have several female and male sexual contacts across the country. They already know the deal—I'm coming through just to let off some stress. I have great dates and companionship with the ladies, and I get my freak on with the brothers when the ladies act up. The brothers are cool because it's always no strings attached. These sisters and brothers are upwardly mobile like I am, so the likelihood of a serious commitment doesn't really enter into the equation.

I started being sexually active with men while I was in graduate school. Back then, I had no interest whatsoever in getting down with a man. I had just dumped this girl I had been dating on and off for a few months and I was feeling a little bad about it. I wanted things to work out, but they didn't.

One of my white buddies went with me to a sports bar to catch a game and talk about women and their trifling ways. We were pretty buzzed, so we took a cab to my place and continued to talk. Eventually, we started talking about sex and sharing war stories. Before long, the conversation just got more detailed about *who* we did and *how* we did it. It was a typical conversation between two men talking about their sexual conquests. But after a few more drinks, the conversation became more open and we both started talking about how freaky we could be.

Unexpectedly, he asked me if I had ever had sex with a man, or ever let a man give me oral sex. I was shocked by his question, but for some reason—probably the loose feeling from the alcohol—I didn't care at this point, and told him no but always wanted to. He told me that he was bisexual and would love to suck me. I gave him his wish and that night was the beginning of my DL lifestyle. After that, I got head from white dudes on a regular basis. I didn't even have to ask for it. It seems that white guys gravitated toward me all the time. Often, I was the first black person they had ever really seen up close.

When they learned I was a grad student, many of them asked if I would be willing to tutor them, and I was down for that. Eventually, "tutoring" came to mean that they wanted to get down with me in some way or another. The arrangement was great because they were really good at sucking my dick and I didn't have to worry about word getting back to my peeps that I was having sex with men. They thought I was getting together with these white guys to study with them.

During this time, I had about three girlfriends. Because of my study schedule, it was easy for me to get out of being with them and connecting with a white guy that was paying me for sex. That way, I had extra money to treat my girlfriends to nice dates and occasional weekend getaways. And I was the perfect gentleman when it came to sex. If she wasn't in the mood for sex or was on her period, it was no problem. I always had a white boy waiting for me.

Leroy shared with me that his life had changed after he read my book, saying that it forced him to take a look at himself. He told me that he didn't want to buy the book, even though it called his name every time he went near a bookstore, and he would avoid going to bookstores, which were his favorite places to go on Saturdays, so he wouldn't have to see it. When he finally purchased it, it stayed in the bag and in the trunk of his BMW for weeks because he didn't want to read it. Then one day he said he opened it up and started to read. Once he began, he couldn't put it down. It was like someone had written his life story. He said as he read he cried. He thought about all the lies and all the shady things he had done to so many women—black, white, Hispanic. He loved women, and had used and abused so many because of his life on the DL.

After he finished the book, he said he sat in his condo for hours. The phone would ring, but he didn't answer it. He was frozen in thoughts that needed his attention. There was no sound in his two-level, 2,500-square-foot home, just his own heart beating. He got on his knees and started praying, asking God for forgiveness and to change him. He had prayed this prayer many times before, and every time he would fall back into the same behavior. But, this time it was different. This time his soul was searching for help. He pleaded with God to allow him to be at peace with himself. He said he asked God that if it was His will for him to be gay, then let him accept it and move on. If it was His will for him to marry a women and have a family, then to please let the desire for men disappear and never return. After this long and sincere talk with God, he got up off his knees, feeling as if a million tons of guilt had been lifted from his shoulders. He opened up the blinds, turned on the stereo, put on his favorite CD, and took a long shower. While he was in the shower, he said it felt like the old him was being washed off and he felt like a new man. He had finally come to a realization that he could no longer use and abuse other humans. He didn't think he would publicly announce he was gay and proud or that he was bisexual, but he would be honest from now on, with himself first, but also with the women he was involved with. He would be up front with any sexual partner and practice a safer sex routine. This was a big step in the right direction. He said that at last he felt free and was finally living a life that gave him peace.

THE GUY NEXT DOOR

This profile is a married man or is in a long-term relationship with a woman. His life doesn't change much from going to work and being at home. This man doesn't cause waves in his life or have drama in his world. He pays his bills and allows his woman to run the household. He goes out with his friends a couple of times per month, and he is often involved in his community.

There is a brother who lives in the same community as I do. He is married with four children, all under ten years old. His wife is a very sweet sister who always speaks to me when she sees me. We have had many conversations about my work and she has asked me many questions about my book. She had seen me on various television shows and read about me. One day she told me that she wanted me to meet some of her girlfriends to have a discussion about my book.

I know her husband through one of my staff members. We would greet each other whenever we bumped into each other but it was very impersonal. One day I ran into him at the drug store. I was in line and he was right behind me. He tapped me on the shoulder and we greeted each other. The line was moving slowly, which gave us the opportunity to talk more than our usual hello. He was a bank officer and he asked me why I wasn't banking at his bank. He teased me about bringing my millions to him to manage for me. We both laughed, and for the first time we connected.

I gave him my cell number and told him that we should get together one day and hang out. Maybe do dinner or go shoot some pool. He said he would be in touch.

Later that week, he called me and asked if I could meet him at the park. I told him to give me about ten minutes and I would meet him near the fountain.

When I arrived he was already sitting there. We shook hands and I sat down and asked him what was up. He said that he needed some advice, but he also needed to know that what he shared with me would stay between us. I agreed. He hesitated for a moment and then said, "I think I'm gay." I looked at him but didn't say a word. I knew there was more he wanted to get off his chest. He wasn't looking at me, but off into the distance. He said that he had been cruising gay websites and that he had met a couple of guys who he allowed to perform oral sex on him. He also had gone to a hotel one afternoon and screwed a man that he'd met online. He said that he used a condom, even when he performed oral sex on the man. But he was concerned that his online activities were getting out of control and he was spending more and more time online looking at personal ads for other brothers on the DL. He had even placed an ad looking to attract DL connections. He knew it was wrong, but he was having a very hard time stopping. He asked me what he should do. He hated himself in the aftermath of all of his hook-ups with men, but at the same time he loved the feeling that being with a man gave him.

We talked about his situation and whether or not he felt comfortable sharing what he was going through with his wife. Although he wanted to talk to her and tell her about his desires, he was afraid that she would leave him and take the children. He said he loved her and didn't want to do anything to hurt her. He had come to me because he had heard his wife talking to her sisters about me and my book. He said he really needed my advice and help.

I told him that the first thing he needed to do was to be honest with himself and come to grips with his bisexuality. I also told him that the only thing that he's doing wrong is cheating on his wife; he always used condoms, even when he was having oral sex, so at least he hadn't placed his wife's health in jeopardy. I asked him if he thought she would leave him if he came clean to her. He didn't know, but he felt he needed her now more than ever. She'd always been his best friend, and they had been through a lot together. He was willing to open up to her, win or lose. He loved her too much to continue to be dishonest with her. Sadly, there are many men who would rather die then confess that they had sex with another women, let alone another man. I told him that he should talk to his pastor if he felt that he would offer good support. And if he needed me to be there I would. We left the park with a commitment that the next time he felt the desires to be with a man, he would call me for support. He also told me that he would talk to his pastor and get his support and then move ahead with talking to his wife.

About a month later I ran into both of them and they looked happy. I called him later that day and asked him what happened. He had told his wife everything and they were trying to work it out. He was getting counseling, and by being able to talk to his wife, he finds he's not so eager to seek out men to have sex. He is more focused on repairing the damage he has put in the relationship with his family and is sincerely trying to keep that family together.

THE URBAN BROTHER

This profile was developed from talking to hundreds of hip-hop-generation men. Some were part of the criminal justice system, and many were living on their own for the first time. Many others were still in college.

Jaymal is a nineteen-year-old freshman at a community college. He has a ten-month-old daughter with his high school girlfriend. In my tour last year I met many young men with similar stories.

Dear Mr. King,

I recently heard that you are going to be in my hometown to speak. I want to meet with you personally to discuss something. I have no one else to talk to about this situation in my life.

I have been having sex with one of the professors at my school. He is thirty-nine years old, married, has twin sons, and lives outside of the city where the college is located.

We get together every day in his office and have sex. I love being with him and we have fun, we laugh, and he helps me with my school projects. I have been to his house for dinner and he even purchased some gifts for my daughter and helped both me and my girlfriend buy a car. He is a nice brother and I respect him and enjoy his company and friendship.

When we have sex, it is so good. He is the bottom and I penetrate him. At first we used condoms, but now we don't. It feels better without them. I know what you are thinking, but that is the way it is.

He recently told me that he loved me, and wanted us to be together. He said that he didn't want to leave his wife, but wanted me to be in his life also. I asked him how we were going to do that, and he said as long as I don't tell anyone about our relationship, and we keep our relationship on the "low," then we can continue doing our thing.

No one knows about us. *No one.* His wife is sweet. She is white. She likes me and always invites me over and tells me to

bring my girlfriend and baby. I don't feel guilty about my relationship with her husband. He is a good father and a wonderful
husband. In fact, I hope to be the same kind of father and husband one day. He is my role model.

My question to you is, should I break this relationship off or
should I continue to be with him? I don't want to break it off. I
feel that I am doing nothing wrong and it would hurt me not to
have him in my life.

Jaymal left me his cell number and asked me to call
him when I got to town. After I checked into my hotel, I
decided to call him. We spoke and I invited him to meet me
for lunch. When he showed up at the Wendy's I was surprised to see how young he looked. He had a baby face,
shoulder-length locks, and a beautiful smile. He looked like
a model. He sat down and we talked. He didn't say much at
first, so I had to take control of the conversation.

I asked him if he'd told anyone that he was meeting
with me. He said no. I asked him if he had decided if he was
going to stay in the relationship with the professor or break
it off. He said that he was undecided, but was leaning more
toward staying in the relationship.

After about an hour of talking, he began to understand
that he was bisexual, and understood what that meant. He
confessed to already thinking that he might be gay, but he
didn't like feeling that way. He hated the out gay men on his
campus. He thought, why would they want everybody to
know their business? Once he understood what being bisexual meant, he said he could accept that and understood why

he had feelings for both the professor and his girlfriend. He asked me if it was fair that his girlfriend didn't know about his sexual orientation. I told him that she should have the choice if she wants to be with a bisexual man, and that he had no right to make that decision for her. He needed to somehow tell her and let her make the decision if she wants to be with him or not.

He was scared and told me that to tell her would be difficult, especially in his small hometown. If the word got out, it would hurt a lot of people and he would not be able to live there anymore. He told me about his uncles and his strong grandfather and how his family was respected. He said that he didn't have anywhere to go, and what would he do about his schooling? His church was paying his tuition and for his books. He said that he had no real job and he didn't want his child to depend on welfare. He knew so many young women in his community were living off government assistance, and he didn't want that for his daughter. These concerns were too great, and he could not put his family and his child at risk to be ruined just because he needed to tell his baby's mother the truth about what he'd been doing and the feelings he had.

I told him I understood, but the least he could do was to make sure that he always protected himself, and make sure that he always knew his HIV status, and make it clear to the professor that even if they stayed on the DL, they would stop putting each other at risk for STDs.

He agreed that he would do that and that he would never again have sex without using a condom out of respect for the other parties involved: his girl, his baby, and also the professor's wife and family.

After we talked, he felt so much better. I think having at least started to have an open conversation about his sexuality was a positive step, perhaps the first to him leading a fully open, honest life with himself and his loved ones. But in the meantime, I was pleased that he was at least going to be safe. If all men who are living on the DL would just do that, then at least a secretive life wouldn't lead to HIV and AIDS spreading to loved ones.

THE MATURE BROTHER

This man has reached a point in his life where he is close to retirement or retired. He has raised his children and has either been married for many years or is a widower who is dating again. He takes good care of himself and feels good about his accomplishments. He also is active in his community and church and has established good friends. I interviewed many ministers who fit into this specific profile.

Noel is a fifty-nine-year-old ex-marine who retired after giving Uncle Sam forty years of his life in the U.S. military. His wife died of cancer about five years ago. He never remarried but dated a lot. Many of the sisters and white women he dated he met at his regular Saturday-night bowling outing. He is a very handsome man, six foot four, well built, and a hint of gray hair in his goatee. He drives a new car and had a very nice home in an upscale community outside of Cleveland, Ohio.

Through his married life, he never messed around with men. He had experienced a couple of blow jobs when he was in the military, but nothing serious, in his mind. He only got oral sex from men when he was away from his wife. He would allow men in the cities or town where he was stationed to suck him off after he left a club. But he never went after any men for more than a quick moment of sexual satisfaction. He was in love with his wife, and he vowed never to divorce or remarry.

Now that he is single and enjoying life, he has decided that he would let his desires to have sex with men come out. At first he was having sex with both the men and women he was seeing. He was living on the DL, but he thought that with men it was just sex, and his emotions were not involved. He was mature, had seen life, traveled around the world, had saved some money, and was doing well for himself. His children are all grown and also doing well. He loved being a grandfather to his eight grandchildren and spending time with them was a joy.

He met a man at a bowling tournament in Louisville, Kentucky. They had a lot in common and ended up exchanging numbers and planned on getting together to go flyfishing. The man, George, was another mature brother in his late forties. Like Noel, he was a successful man who was comfortable with his life, though he was in the process of getting a divorce. When they went on their fly-fishing trip they picked a remote location in the hills of Kentucky, where the fishing was known to be excellent. It was just the two of them. Prior to this meeting, neither one talked about sexual orientation or if they "messed" around. They just enjoyed each other's company and vibed well with each other. Both men were seeking a male friend to do things with.

During the weekend, they got a chance to talk about their past and what they wanted in life. Noel felt that this man really understood him and he wanted to share with him that he was bisexual. At first he was nervous because he didn't want to lose a good friend, but he didn't want to live a lie with this man. He wanted him to know him for who he is. He wanted him to accept him for being comfortable with being bisexual and make it clear to him that he was not holding back his feelings for men. In fact, he was really attracted to George and wanted him to know it.

The last night of their trip, Noel decided to tell George that he was attracted to him and he would like for them to be more then just friends.

As they were cooking over an open fire, Noel told George everything: about his dearly departed wife, his beautiful adult children, and his angelic grandchildren. He also told him that he was bisexual, and at this time of his life, he wanted to see if he could fall in love with a man and create a relationship.

George listened to him, and after he was finished told him that he also was bisexual and had lived his life on the DL. He had developed a secret sex life with other men behind his wife's back. He told Noel that he was tired of lying to his friends and family. Now he wanted just to be who he was. But he knew that he couldn't be out about his sexuality. His biggest reason was his position with his church.

The two of them agreed that they would get to know each other and promised that they would not have sex with other people while they were figuring out their own relationship. They would be each other's support system. Despite the ways in which they'd both lived DL in the past, they were sure they didn't want to go on that way. Both of them were fathers of daughters and didn't want their loved ones to have to deal with men who were still living a lie and hurting others.

Noel told me that for him to be able to tell another brother about his sexuality made him feel as if he'd finally exhaled. It felt good to have someone in his life that accepted him for him and could understand what a confusing road he had traveled.

This is the pot of gold at the end of the rainbow for so many men and women struggling to come up from the DL: the exhilarating liberation that comes from emerging from behind a cloud of lies to finally live the truth.

5

MOVING PAST THE DOWN LOW

J ames Baldwin once wrote that one of the important
lessons he learned while growing up on the streets
of Harlem was to always walk toward the thing you
fear. It took courage to stare danger in the face, but
he knew it would be a bigger mistake to turn his back on it.
This is a lesson we can all use: When faced with a difficult
situation, face it head on. I offer this advice to anyone who
is forced to deal with any kind of difficult situation or negative behavior. Face it head on and deal with it. This applies
to individuals, families, and even whole communities.

Having met so many DL men and heard them share
the full range of their emotions—from pain to arrogance,
from greed and lust to insecurity and self-hatred—I feel in
my heart that these men are in no way proud of their behavior and fear being exposed to their loved ones. Yes, by living
DL their desires are being fed, but they are hurting themselves
and others in the process. When their behavior is revealed it

often comes at a great cost, but at least their life on the down low no longer exists. Once out in the open, they're forced to deal with the consequences of what they've done and answer a lot of questions to both their loved ones and themselves. When a DL person comes forward they are disrupting not only their companion's life, but many other people in their immediate circle. An entire community can often feel the fall-out of a single person's selfishness and confusion.

In addition to meeting so many DL men, I've also heard the stories of many people who are part of the larger community. Not just the deceived spouses, but also the friends, other family members, pastors, and professional colleagues of the DL man. Many of them have told me that just because they discover the DL man's true sexual identity, it doesn't mean they stop loving that person.

My relationship with my exwife is a good example of how a couple can heal and move on with their lives. We worked on our relationship, and with prayer and communication we were eventually able to restore the respect we once had for each other. I was able to learn how to be myself with her—my true self—and she was able to forgive me and move on. That is the main reason I encouraged her to write her story. I felt that her story was needed to give an insider's perspective of how DL behavior affects the spouses and lovers for whom it's a stinging act of betrayal. But I also thought she'd give an insider's perspective on how even that kind of cutting betrayal can be forgiven and the relationship redeemed.

But at the time my marriage fell apart, I was devastated. And not just because I'd lost my wife, but because I was lost to a whole community of friends, family, and faith. I ended up leaving town altogether to avoid facing the pain. I started a new life but still had my DL ways. In my new life, in my new town, I met new women who had no idea who I was. To them, I was just the new sharp, well-dressed, handsome bachelor in town. But inside I was an ugly mess, completely hideous to myself. I was on a horrible destructive path. I hated myself. I wanted to kill myself. But I also thought that taking my life would give me an instant ticket to hell. My belief in God wouldn't let me do it. I was smoking, drinking, and recklessly spending my money. I was still lying to the women I'd in various ways committed myself to, still having sex with both men and women. If I was having sex with one woman, then I was having sex with six men. And then when I'd come home from having sex with a stranger I'd be over-whelmed by feelings of disgust. I was beating myself up, but I still couldn't stop. I now know that I was not alone in my behavior.

The fact is that I was ultimately responsible for my ill behavior. I'm the one who allowed confusion and desire to lead me into a self-destructive and damaging lifestyle. At the same time, I was in some ways pinned in by the community I was surrounded by. First I was pressured into trying to pass myself off as completely heterosexual so as not to find myself banished from the community. When I was DL, I felt robbed of all the resources I'd depended on my whole life:

my family, my friends, my church. I was alone and haunted, which only increased my recklessness. Then, when the facts were out, I felt I had no choice but to exile myself from home. The cycle of depression and loneliness only made my DL behavior worse and more persistent. The fact is that without community support, DL behavior is only aggravated and made worse. From the very first stages, before it reaches the destructive, suicidal point it reached with me, the overall community needs to make it clear to an individual that he has choices with regards to his sexuality and doesn't need to suppress his natural feelings or only let them out in secrecy, where they'll do the most damage. The community as a whole—and that means all of us—needs to open wide the door to acceptance, which will only make it easier for people to explore honestly and openly their own sexuality.

The African American church and African American fraternities reach millions of black men. If these respected institutions would provide education and support to men regardless of sexual orientation, then the battle against DL behavior and all of its attendant ills (meaning its role in destroying relationships and in spreading HIV) would be considerably easier.

There are also other organizations that can do their part: the Masonic Fraternal Order of Brotherhood, the Prince Hall Masons, national social groups like the 100 Black Men and many others. If everyone came together with one message, the power and impact it would make would reach millions. As of now, these organizations are slow to open themselves to black men who have nonheterosexual identities and, as a result, force their members to make a choice: either live as a visibly straight person or lose your role in our organization, which has been providing you with friendship, support, outlets for community service, and professional contacts. It's a very difficult choice for most men to make.

The church is another case altogether. As a man raised in the black church, the fear of God was put in me from as early as I can remember. Growing up, I remember hearing pastors talking about how God will use His power to strike down anyone who isn't living righteous, which to some pastors means following the Ten Commandants and the rest of the laws given in the Bible in a literal sense, word for word. The church I grew up in is like a lot of black churches across the country: When it came to sexual sins in particular, they didn't play. I have seen pregnant girls that I grew up with forced to stand up at the front of the church and ask for forgiveness for being "too fast." It was shameful for her and her family. And that kind of shame exerts a real coercive pressure on the members of the congregation, which in some cases leads them to do whatever it is they can to avoid having their "sins" revealed in public. I remember another young girl who got pregnant but wore a girdle because her parents didn't want anyone to know that she was with child.

The kinds of churches I came up in could be chilling places for someone who felt sin lurking within him. I can still hear the deacons and the mothers in the church singing at the top of their lungs that "soon and very soon/we are going to see the King." And then hear my father, himself a longtime deacon, say, "In the by and by we all will walk the streets of gold, and everybody will stand before God and be judged." These messages scared the hell out of me. I took it so seriously that I was sure if I went to a movie on a Sunday I would go to hell. If I cussed, I just knew I would end up in the fiery furnace and burn forever. I was so shaken up by all of the talk of God and the devil and evil spirits that I was scared to sleep in the dark. I didn't want God to come and get me because I was thinking naughty thoughts or having wet dreams about that brother in the youth choir. "Man, why me Lord, why me?" I would ask myself.

I tried to read the scriptures to get an understanding of what it is that God wanted from me. I heard that a man who finds a wife is blessed. I heard that when I gave my life to Christ and got baptized that I came out of the sacred water a new man; the old man was washed white as snow. But some things didn't change, even after I was baptized. I still wanted to go to the movies on Sunday and listen to "the devil's music." I still wanted to get with the brother in the choir, and I still was having wet dreams about having sex with men that I had seen or met. Was there no hope for my soul? I felt doomed—even worse, I felt damned.

Those feelings stayed with me for 99 percent of my adult life. Even now I haven't completely shaken them. People sometimes want to talk to me about my spiritual life.

They ask, "Do you have a personal relationship with God? Do you really think you're lifestyle is acceptable by God? Do you think you're getting into heaven even though you have sex with men?" When I hear those questions, sometimes I wonder: Maybe God is going to send me to the deepest pits of hell.

It's just that kind of fear that keeps many men on the DL and scared to come out. Scared, first of all, to come out and face the judgment of the church. But also scared to come out to themselves, even in the privacy of their own minds, because of what the church has instilled in them about just how sinful and abominable homosexual behavior is. As far as the church goes, these men know that folks will just shake their heads and pass whatever personal judgments they want. But to some, in their minds, they are more concerned that they will actually end up in hell. In many black communities God is presented as this vengeful being who hates all wrongdoing but reserves a special hatred for people who are not heterosexual, as if premarital sex or adultery with someone of the same sex is any worse than those same sins committed with someone of the opposite sex.

So as a result, at many churches no one talks about these forms of sexuality. No one talks about the bisexual, gay, and lesbian brothers and sisters that are filling the pews every Sunday. At some churches, no one even wants to talk about the epidemic of general promiscuity—including heterosexual adultery—that's tearing up families and helping to spread HIV/AIDS. It's all kept on the hush-hush, as if by not speaking its name it will somehow go away. But how can we ever win the battle against HIV/AIDS, adultery, and homophobia if we don't want to accept that they exist? How will we provide education, information, and support to people who are hurting if we can't agree that there is a problem? When will men who feel that they have nothing to do with the spread of HIV because they are not gay or on the DL step up and do their part? Why won't more churches take a leadership role in helping to calm growing fears about the DL phenomenon by admitting that homosexual and bisexual members are active in church leadership and should be accepted for who they are, regardless of their sexual behavior?

These are questions that I ask myself every day. And I have sought answers from community leaders, pastors, and close associates who I respect. There is a division on this issue in the African American church. Some churches are doing some great work in providing HIV education to their community and working to eliminate homophobia. But many are still preaching messages of hate and not doing anything to heal their members and provide support to their community.

For instance, my friend Bishop Keith Brian Williams, pastor of the All Nations Church in Columbus, Ohio, believes that the first step for any church is to be honest about itself. He writes in his book, *Ministering Graciously to the Gay and Lesbian Community,* "Though I am a straight man, married to my wife for over twenty-five years, and though I have always been straight, I have members of my extended family that have struggled with same-sex attraction. I also have many very dear friends in the ministry and in business who either were or are gay or lesbian. I have many parishioners that I have pastored whose lives have been checkered with this proclivity and I am acquainted with a number of public, civic, and church leaders who daily lead a duplicitous lifestyle. If the truth be told, this sad fact is a more common occurrence than most people are ready to acknowledge and admit. I believe that whenever you tell the truth that you shame the devil."

I admire and respect the ministry of Dr. Jeremiah A. Wright, Jr., pastor of Trinity UCC located on the south side of Chicago. Dr. Wright's primary message is that no one sin is greater than another sin. He doesn't preach that the sin of homosexuality is greater than any other sexual sin. Nor have I ever heard him tell his congregation that homosexuality is a one-way ticket to hell. There are SGL ministries for his homosexual members, and he allows them to hold leadership roles in the church and does not make them feel separate from the other members. His huge congregation of more than 15,000 members is affirming and welcome to all sexual orientations. I have met other pastors around the country who are doing their part to provide information and education to their community, with the goal of holding families and communities together, giving them a chance to have more weddings than funerals.

I also have met many outspoken pastors who have

stepped past what their members will accept and give them the message that they feel they need to hear, whether they like it or not. Many of these men and women have put their own position in jeopardy because they have invited me to speak at their church, or they have not folded to the pressure of those in the church who only want one message when it comes to homosexuality: that it is a sin and an abomination. These pastors deserve special credit for being in the vanguard of change, even at personal risk.

I have been invited to speak at over a dozen African American churches as part of their health-fair events or HIV prevention programs. Because they know that none of their DL men would step up and speak about their own lives, many pastors invite me to come in and speak about the behavior and give a message that will reach their male members. These events are well received when the pastor sets the tone prior to the event, but telling the men in the congregation how important it is for them to be leaders in the church and not sit back and let their community die off because of silence and shame. One of those pastors, David L. Ferguson, pastor of the First AME Church, Altamonte Springs, Florida, agreed to share some of what he's learned here.

What is the church's role in providing support to gay and bisexual men?

My personal view of this might not line up with my peers, but there should be no distinction in the support given to gay and bisexual men and the support shown to straight men or women. We are all equal in God's eyes, although varied or nontraditional lifestyles might produce a unique set of circumstances and challenges to the leadership of the church. In the church, an issue is an issue and those who struggle with any issues are still members of the congregations, giving tithes, helping to support the various ministries within the church, so they deserve no less support from the church just because they live a lifestyle that is not yet completely socially acceptable.

What is the church's role in providing HIV education to the community?

Within the church community, we must take an active stand and a solidified position with respect to educating our communities about the spread of HIV. The purpose of the church is to administer to the needs of the community in which it is based, and even beyond, if the opportunity presents itself. There is a definite need to educate on HIV in our community. We cannot allow society to dictate to the church which needs it should be administering to. If the church goes about it the right way, it should be an example to society of how we should treat others that are in need. Too many churches have allowed societal opinions to infiltrate the meaning and the purpose of real ministry.

Why do you think pastors who live on the DL won't be examples and come clean about their personal lives?

Again, I can only offer my opinion on this matter. I have no practical experience to support my view on the subject, but I do believe that a DL pastor is like a pastor who gambles, drinks, or fraternizes with women. Whether we as pastors like it or not, we are examples to our congregation. Unfortunately, wearing a collar does not exempt us from public ridicule and scrutiny. In fact, being in the ministry makes you more vulnerable to criticism. Because of this fact, many pastors who may be on the DL will not come clean about their lifestyle. The truth of the matter is that people are not looking for positive things to spread about the pastor, but they look for negative things to spread. In our society, a pastor doing right or "good" is not news because it is the expectation of the calling, but when a pastor violates the expectations of society, people want to hear about that. Unfortunately, we have allowed society to influence our ability to exert influence in the community. Because most pastors depend on the church for their livelihood, they also have to be cognizant of the fact that most church members frown on DL behavior. To put it plainly, "The hand that feeds you, controls you."

What is your message to men who are having sex with men and not telling their female partners?

A woman, or any sexual partner, has the right to know if they are being put at risk by having sex with someone who is practicing sexual relations with another individual. Although there should be a certain amount of discretion and privacy afforded our sexual partners, there is also a moral obligation that we as men have with respect to the physical and emotional well-being of the women in our lives. The Bible says that we are to love our neighbors as ourselves. In doing so, we must ask ourselves the question, "Would we want to be treated in the same manner in which we treat our women?" Sex is something to be shared between two people as an expression of love and a means to reproduce. I don't know that there is a foundation of love as it relates to two men being sexually involved while one man is actively involved with a woman as well, but I do know that it is not for the purpose of reproducing offspring. Having said that, it is incumbent upon men to advise a woman that he is having sex with another man.

What is your message to the community as it pertains to sex, sexuality, and sexual behavior?

Sex is something that we have got to recognize and accept as a common part of our culture. I don't say that to be cavalier about sex, but we can't continue to converse about sex only behind "closed doors." To continue to avoid speaking about something as prevalent and potentially life altering as sex is tantamount to denying the existence of it.

I'm not referring to sexual behavior as it relates to specific sexual acts, but as the respect and consideration that is due our partners. Our sexual behavior needs to be tied to our idea of love, safety, and morality along with our virtues.

As for the pastors who have come up from the down low themselves, these pastors are proof that we are weak and sometimes fall short. One of these former DL pastors agreed

COMING UP FROM THE DOWN LOW

to share some of his opinions and history here. This brother is now a pastor of a church in Tampa, Florida. He lives as an openly gay man who is in a committed relationship with a man. He is the father of a grown daughter and is one of the most spiritual men I know. I asked the pastor how he was able to leave his former down-low life and come out to his family and friends about his sexual orientation. This is what he had to say.

As an openly gay father and pastor, what is your opinion of men on the DL?

"And ye shall know the truth, and the truth shall set you free . . ." says it all. Most DL men operate in a mood of deceit and that troubles me from the perspective that they're captive to their lies. For me, it's a sad state when someone has to live a lie; eventually it becomes their truth, and the line between truth and deceit becomes the proverbial thin—if not invisible—line. That web of deceit begins to entangle and then endanger the lives of others. I think it's important that brotha's free themselves from the lies, define who they are clearly and publicly, and not operate in this mode of deceit.

What do you think is needed to bring healing in the black community as it pertains to this DL issue?

Understanding. There is still such confusion where this issue is concerned. Most people see this as a gay man in denial, and for some that may be the truth. For others gender is not an issue, but bisexual doesn't define it either. The African American community is a no-gray-area kind of community, and for them it's either you are or you aren't. Again, the whole DL phenomenon isn't anything new; it's the definition and classification that people are having a hard time wrapping their brains around.

What do you tell your straight minister friends when they only want to preach hatred against homosexuality?

I remind them of the account in the Bible where a woman is caught in adultery and brought before Jesus. He doesn't condemn her to hell or put her on blast for her sins. Instead he challenges her accusers with the statement, "Ye that is without sin cast the first stone." Sin is sin and will always be, but it's the sinner who stands needing the same compassion from you that the woman received from Jesus. If we're going call ourselves Christians and be Christ-like, then shouldn't we try to be like Christ? I ask them about the people involved in ministry at their church: are there gay or those perceived as gay actively involved in their choirs, performing arts ministry, etc.? And a great majority of the time they tell me yes. My comment to them then is that if these people are active in their ministry and if the pastors encourage their participation and then blast them from the pulpit, they're hypocrites.

What do you tell DL men who seek out counseling to deal with their struggles with their sexuality?

Ralph Ellison says, "When I discover who I am, I'll be free" and I think that it's imperative to men on the down low to really discover who they are. Whether they're bisexual or gay or even men who don't care, they still need to acknowledge who they are in order to become who they are. If they're ever going

COMING UP FROM THE DOWN LOW

to live in their truth, it's about leaving the lies behind. It's about living a life free of the deceit and plotting, manipulation and selfish behavior.

What was your conversation like with your daughter when you told her you were gay?

I didn't get to tell my daughter that I was gay. My exwife did. I didn't find out until a few years later that she already knew. I was very angry that my exwife took it upon herself to tell my daughter her version of "your dad likes men." I must say, much to my daughter's credit, she didn't miss a beat. She reaffirmed that I'm still her father regardless and that she was proud to be my daughter.

There are other levels of community besides the church that can take more of an active leadership role in promoting awareness of the DL lifestyle and opening the way for people to live in a freer way. I often wondered why Black fraternities are not dealing with homosexuality in their organizations or establishing stronger HIV prevention programs for their members. I love where the black Greek sororities are when it comes to providing HIV programming and making sure that their members are aware and informed. But I have never been invited to speak to at Alpha's, Kappa's, Q's, Sigma's, or any African-American male organization's national conferences or conventions. In fact, I don't know anyone who has addressed the issues of sexual orientation to the black Greek organizations. Many leaders know that that they have gay and bisexual members but don't want to accept it. It is a perfect example of "don't ask, don't tell." I have been told by many of my friends that their fraternities will never accept that they have gay or DL members.

I wanted to know why this attitude exists when I know so many DL men who are in fraternities. I asked Dr. Walter M. Kimbrough, vice president of student affairs at Albany State University in Albany, Georgia, and author of *Black Greek 101* about the reason fraternities are not accepting that this behavior is very much a part of the lifestyle of many of their members. This is what he had to say:

Many leaders know that they have gay and bisexual members but don't want to accept it. It is a perfect example of "don't ask, don't tell." Why does this attitude exist?

I think black fraternities are just a microcosm of black America—we're homophobic. The issue is even more of a touchy subject with fraternities because over the years they have been able to see their gay brothers coming out more openly, and I know this makes many members very uncomfortable. Fraternities and sororities reinforce the heterosexual nature of America, so anything that differs from that becomes difficult to accept. I think this has been why we have seen gay fraternities emerge in the last twenty years—the largest is Delta Lambda Phi, but that's basically a white fraternity. A black gay fraternity was started at Florida State in the late 1980s, but I don't believe it is functioning today.

What do you think fraternities can do to bring HIV/AIDS education and awareness to the members?

For prevention, I think that the fraternities have to make HIV/AIDS a real issue to their members without making it seem like their "manhood" is being challenged. There is the fact that HIV/AIDS can be gotten through heterosexual contact as well, and because they're trying to maintain a hyper-macho image, many of the members like to brag about their sexual conquests. So that is definitely a way to get them interested in HIV/AIDS and the DL issue. Also, I think the DL issue can be raised because these men could be having sex with women who are having sex with DL men, so that may be another way to address the issue. Although it is possible for this kind of consciousness raising to occur, the leaders of the fraternities need to be approached by a broad coalition of health providers to address it. Also, they all have members who work actively in terms of HIV/AIDS and they can provide leadership as well. I do know that on some local and state levels, HIV/AIDS is a topic and issue that fraternities deal with.

I have many gay and bisexual friends who belong to Greek organizations who feel that they would be ostracized, blacklisted, or even harmed if they were to make their sexual orientation known. What would you tell them?

I would tell them that they can come out to open-minded brothers, and over time I have hope that the organizations will be more open-minded. In many ways, as I have indicated, all the fraternities clearly know they have gay members, so it might not be as controversial as some might think. I think that if someone in leadership within a fraternity, like a president or vice president, ever came out, it would be a good role model for others. It may be easier if a coalition of gay men representing all of the fraternities came out together to show that it isn't just one group, but all of them, then maybe we could address the issue.

I think that for college men, many are trying to develop their own identity, so coming out is even tougher. We know that in recent years gay college students have been murdered. Fraternity men are very afraid of being labeled as a "gay" frat, and will often overcompensate and go straight gangster to get away from that image. As an undergraduate, my chapter always voted no on anyone thought to be "suspect," because a few years earlier some chapter members were either known or thought to be gay. So we definitely began bringing in men who were ladies' men and known for their conquests. I see this dynamic happening with all fraternities on campuses today.

I have met many doctors who have shared their expertise about HIV prevention. These professionals work daily with patients and provide care to many people who are HIV positive or have AIDS.

I have been on many panels with doctors who reveal what they are seeing from their patients who come in and test for HIV. One young doctor told me that he always has young black men who test HIV positive, and when he asks them how do they think they got infected, most don't give him an answer. When he asked them if they had been sexually involved with another man, all of them tell him no. Even when he suspects they are lying, they look at him and tell him no, they're not gay and don't have sex with men. He told me once that he would like to understand more about this DL behavior. If he could understand it, maybe he could help his male clients, especially since he works at an inner-city urban clinic where nearly 100 percent of his clients are African American.

During my initial speaking engagements, my audiences would come to me looking for specific health information. It's a testament to the discomfort that many black people feel toward healthcare professionals that they would come to me, a layman, to get health advice. My friend Dr. David Malebranche, M.D., M.P.H., and assistant professor of Emory University, Division of General Medicine, Atlanta, Georgia, told me that I should allow those who work in public health to join me at any speaking engagements so they can give specific medical advice and current data about HIV/AIDS. I can then freely talk about the behavior and give my HIV prevention message—practice safer sex and honesty. I've been invited to speak at medical conferences and before federal agencies for my expertise in this subject; but I also know my limits.

I wanted you to hear from doctors who can provide insight about the current trends about the spread of HIV. I have learned a lot spending time with these dedicated physicians, and it is important that all of us get a clear understanding about this disease, since it is ravaging our community. We need to know our enemy so we can stop it before it annihilates us.

One of the things to be aware of, however, is that there are active debates going on between medical professionals. In particular, there are physicians, like Dr. Coleman-Miller, who I cited earlier, who believe that the DL phenomenon *is* a contributing factor to the expansion of HIV among women. Others believe that the DL is overstated as a factor. It's hard to tell where science ends and political ideas begin; just as some people love the idea of scapegoating DL men for the rise in HIV/AIDS, others are trying to let DL men off the hook altogether. Both extremes seem motivated by political concerns: one motivated by homophobia, the other by a desire to counter homophobia. So it's important to hear both sides of the issue. I wanted to include here the voice of a physician who argues that the causes for the rise in HIV/AIDS among black women has a multitude of causes. I disagree with some of his reasoning, but most of what he says is of great value. One key point: It's unfair to scapegoat DL men for the rise in HIV. Another key point is that the DL is symptomatic of larger problems of sexual confusion and irresponsibility in our communities that we all need to be honest about and confront.

The current focus on the "down low" in the black community has successfully opened the doors to conversation regarding sexual behavior, sexual identity, and our communication and testing practices. However, the down side is that this fruitful conversation has often been peppered with overexaggerated and inaccurate portrayals of black men as guilty bisexual predators

COMING UP FROM THE DOWN LOW

and black heterosexual women as innocent uninformed victims. Not only are these portrayals not entirely true, but they're leading us into an unproductive discussion of HIV blame in our community that refuses to address the complexity of this issue.

From many behavioral research studies, we know that black men are less likely to identify as "gay" and more likely to be behaviorally bisexual than white men, despite engaging in homosexual behavior. Black men are also less likely to disclose their homosexual behavior to friends, family, and coworkers than white men. While this is interesting to discuss and often leads people into knee-jerk conclusions that black men are full of "internalized homophobia" and self-hatred due to religious beliefs, notions of masculinity, and mental health, we must remain clear that these findings do not necessarily predict HIV status or risky sexual behavior. In fact, there is evidence that black men who adopt a "gay identity" and disclose their homosexual behavior to others are actually more likely to be HIV positive and engage in unprotected anal sex than those who don't. What we hear in the media about secretive bisexual men is that because so-called down-low men are secretive about their sexual behavior with both genders, they engage in unprotected sex more than those who are open about their sexuality. This is not true, and flies against the political gay-rights movement that proposes that homosexual men will engage in safer sex if they just "come out of the closet." While this may be true for white men, it is certainly not the case for black men. Add to this the fact that most of the research on black homosexual men has found high rates of HIV among those who are "gay-identified," and you'll see the problem America is having with confusing anecdotal cases with public health reports.

The other angle to this "down low" conversation that is often left unaddressed is the role of black women's choice with regards to sexual behavior. We know from current research that black women are engaging in high rates of unprotected anal and vaginal sex, have high rates of sexually transmitted diseases, and douche frequently, all of which may facilitate HIV transmission. Additionally, we know that issues of power, finances, and a shallow pool of available black men may also drive choices to engage in unprotected sex despite adequate knowledge of HIV risk. So why is it that we are not talking more about gender-specific life strategies for black women that engage and empower them to facilitate discussions of HIV risk with their partners, negotiate condom use when considering sexual intercourse, and improve their life circumstances so that they won't be caught in a situation where they have to place immediate life priorities (food, water, shelter, love) over a perceived "long-term" priority such as unprotected sex and acquiring HIV? This question is a difficult one to answer but suggests that the general American public would much rather tell black women that black men are to blame for all their problems (including HIV) instead of encouraging some level of personal responsibility about the larger life issues that influence their sexual behavior.

What it all comes down to is that our HIV prevention strategies in this country have traditionally been flawed, and continue to be flawed in our thinking that HIV can be prevented or slowed down by targeting risk groups instead of risk behaviors. Targeting "down low" brothers for HIV prevention will be a colossal waste of public health time, personnel, and money, because : (1) black men are not the only ethnic group to have HIV or be secretive about their sexual behavior; (2) secrecy

COMING UP FROM THE DOWN LOW

about the gender of one's sexual partners does not mean that one is automatically irresponsible about condom use; and (3) it will give a false sense of security to those who aren't "down low" that they can engage in unprotected sex without worry of risk.

The truth of the matter is that sexual networks among people are extensive and cross racial, ethnic, geographic, class, religious, and political lines. To address this, our HIV-prevention strategies to public health officials and medical providers must focus on the behaviors that are most risky for HIV: unprotected anal and vaginal sex. For medical providers and community based personnel who do HIV screening, this means asking the forty-three-year-old white married woman if she engages in anal sex. The assumption that someone who is white, female, married, and heterosexual is not engaging in anal sex and is not at HIV risk is crazy in this day and age. The sad reality is that with so many people still having unprotected sex and so many with HIV or other STDs, regardless of personal or marriage status, the only person whose sexual behavior you can account for is your own. And the level of risk you are willing to engage in will depend on how well you think you know and trust your sexual partners, both casual and steady. So those of us on the front line of HIV-prevention work need to drop targeting identities such as "bisexual," "heterosexual," and "gay," and focus rather on engaging people in honest dialogue about their individual risk based on what they've been doing sexually, not by what label they call themselves in front of you or others. And all of us in the general community need to take inventory and be honest about our real HIV risk based on our sexual behaviors, not based on denial or image of how we want people to see us.

The message should be simple—if you are engaging in

unprotected anal or vaginal sex, you are at risk for HIV and should be tested. People get tripped up because despite knowing how HIV is transmitted, they don't see themselves at risk because they don't belong to "risk groups." The current risk group du jour is the so-called down-low black men. But we don't have any research to prove this, and it does nothing but further divide a black community that is already divided enough. We don't need to pit black men against black women, black homosexuals against heterosexuals, and black bisexuals against the world—we have a deadly disease that is severely affecting our entire community more so than any other racial/ethnic group in the United States. If we don't start thinking about this epidemic on a more community and global level outside of the "down low," we will be playing this blaming game until we dig ourselves a collective early grave. HIV is quickly becoming genocide for the black community—not because of where it came from, but because of how we're reacting to it now.

This is a compelling argument, but does nothing to undercut the urgency of understanding what's going on with DL men. One major source of confusion about the DL is thinking of it as the primary problem when it comes to HIV transmission when in fact it's just a symptom of the problem. That problem is the combination of ignorance, irresponsibility, and denial that afflicts all of our sexual relationships. If we *all* learn to be open, honest, and responsible about all aspects of our sexual lives, we can lick HIV. At the same time, the DL phenomenon, as the doctor above mentioned, is real, and it cannot be dismissed as a factor, among many, in the rise of HIV transmission. Being responsible about sex means understanding where all of your sexual partners are coming from, in terms of their habits and pasts. While DL men should never be accused or scapegoated as the cause of the HIV explosion in the black community, they also shouldn't be given a free pass for increasing the amount of sexual deception and irresponsibility in our communities, the very attitudes that have fed the epidemic.

6

WOMEN SPEAK OUT

In my travels I have encountered some amazing people with amazing stories. I have been invited to every major city in every state in the country to speak about the Down Low. I have received thousands of e-mails from all over the world, from Africa to Jamaica to Germany. I had no idea that the world was going to respond to my book the way they have. It has been incredible. The range of emotions I've observed in audiences has included sadness, relief, confusion, anger, forgiveness, curiosity, and blame.

In 2004 I did more than 110 DL awareness presentations. I also did more than 52 book signings across the country. At many of my presentations, there was a Q&A at the end, giving the audience an opportunity to ask me questions. There were many times that I did not want to answer questions from the floor because I would open myself up for personal questions. Yes, people have asked me everything under the heavens, from "Are you a top or a bottom" to

"How big is your penis." There is not one question that has not been asked. It got so out of control that I decided to pass out index cards before my presentation, and then later selected the best questions during the Q&A. That way, I could filter out any question that crossed the line.

On my website, I had a message board that provided people with a platform to post their comments or questions. Due to many messages that were offensive to me, other visitors to the board, and my family, I have since shut it down. But I would like to thank the people who shared their stories and gave me their support and prayers. I knew from the start that I would invoke emotions from all different people, but I did not know how many people would share them with me.

What I call the "information gap" when it comes to our sexuality is real and has never been more clear to me than when I read these posts. There's a desperate need for people to find a forum through which they can air their concerns and questions, but also for all of us to share ideas and experiences about the sexuality in an open, nonjudgmental fashion. This is why so many people get in touch with me on a regular basis—and also why I'm sharing some of their experiences and questions here now.

Mr. King,

I wanted to inform you that I recently received an e-mail about DL brothers. I wanted to thank you for the insight you have given. I have to admit, it makes me wonder about the men in my life.

I have been contemplating starting a relationship with a renowned single pastor and I wanted to know how I can test him to see if he is a DL brother, and no, he doesn't have any feminine tendencies. He has expressed interest in me, and I too am interested in him, but I need to know. Now, do not get me wrong, I am seeking the Lord about this matter, but I also know that God gave us each common sense.

Please reply!

In all of this experience of talking publicly about the DL, one of the most disturbing things is the degree to which my comments about a handful of black men, a small subculture, got blown out of proportion. Many women are living in fear because of all the media attention to DL behavior. I think it is great that many women who would have never questioned a man's sexual behavior are now thinking about it and in turn changing their behavior, but I don't think it is healthy for women to live in constant fear to the point where they're afraid that *every* man they encounter is potentially on the DL. As a result, a lot of brothers are being unfairly accused of creeping. But before we dismiss this sister as paranoid, let's remember a few things: she wrote that there didn't seem to be any outward feminine tendencies, but as I discussed earlier, that kind of "sign" is irrelevant. Something is clearly bothering her about this man, even though to the world he seems as straight as an arrow. What should she do?

There's really nothing to do except to have a frank, open conversation about their sexual desires and histories *before* they become intimate. If she can establish an open, nonaccusatory, loving conversational space where they can both feel free to express all of their concerns about sex, then there's a stronger chance that the truth will be revealed than if she goes straight at him with a slew of accusations with no evidence. But when your intuition is tingling, it should at least provide you with motivation to clear the air in a friendly, loving way.

> I read your article and came to your site. I first heard about you by an e-mail that was sent to me from my sister. Since then, I have been writing articles and posting them on various sites to spread the word about men on the down low. I even had a big debate about it in some forums. I'm hurt at the conditions that our black men are in. But I'm also hurt at the lack of respect that black women receive from black men in general. It's like, *damn,* is this what my eleven-year-old daughter has to look forward to, J.L.? I know I probably won't get a response back from you because I can see that you are a busy man. But being black and living in this country is pointless. I just said the other day that if my relationship with my man, an African American brotha, does not work out, I'm done with African American men. I'm not going to jump to the white man either, but no brother from the U.S. will ever get a shot at being with me again. I feel that black women in this nation don't get the respect and honesty that we deserve. If we are not bitches and hoes, we're getting picked over for another man or a white women. And that is real.

I receive a lot of messages of this sort from women who seem to be lost in despair and ready to give up on black men out of a sense of hopelessness. But I take care to make this point as often as I can: *Not all black men are on the DL.* There are still many fine, respectful, hard-working brothers out there who shouldn't be painted with this broad brush. If women object to all black women being reduced to bitches and hoes—as they should—then they should give brothers the same respect by not assuming that all of them are either good-for-nothing, out for white women, or on the DL.

That said, I also think she makes a powerful point, even if she did so unintentionally. For many black women, the DL phenomenon is not really the reason that they have trouble finding a good black man, but they think of it as the final straw. The solution is not blaming DL men, but for all black men to really step up to the challenge of turning ourselves into better mates for our women. DL behavior is not the only reason that many women don't trust men. For years, black men have been portrayed as being uncaring, irresponsible, in prison, on drugs, babymakers who don't take care of their children, or only on the hunt for white women (or any non-black women). Everyday black women read about the lack of black men who are worthy to be with, or they have conversations that end up as "male bashing," which just creates a tough environment for even good black men to be given a chance. Society, family, and friends all play a role on why all black men are being grouped as being not worthy. We need to stop downing all black men and start promoting and celebrating black men who are doing the right thing and looking for love with black women. The kind of despair and hopelessness among black women expressed by the sister above is dangerous—we can't have a whole generation of black women giving up on black men.

> Good morning Mr. King,
>
> I'm emailing you just to say thank you. I just finished reading your book, I was in a coma state. I'm a victim of the DL man and it has ruined my life forever. I've been HIV positive for thirteen years now because of who I loved and cared for and trusted. He let me down. Now after reading your book I see that all the signs were there for me to see.
>
> I was bitter toward men for some time now and I hated most men and wished them all dead. Because of what happened to me I never wanted to see another black man again. I have since gotten over the fact that I am HIV positive and I am doing the same kind of work that you do. I work at a hospital where I educate HIV patients and teach them how to be safer and go on with their everyday life.
>
> After reading your book, I can now say that I no longer hate black men and I have opened my eyes and started to trust again.
>
> I would like to say something to all DL brothers out there: Tell your lady about your lifestyle and give her a chance to decide if she wants to be in a relationship with someone who is bisexual.
>
> Thank you for your words. You have changed my life.

I love the way this sister took something that was a negative in her life and turned it into a positive message to educate and help others so they don't get hurt. The key to moving on is to forgive and don't let the past eat up your life. When you are infected with HIV, it's not going anywhere. You can either learn to live with it, or you can let it eat you up. It is a fact that thinking negative thoughts and holding on to negative feelings only further weaken your immune system and open you up to other sicknesses. Love is a powerful thing, and it can make even the hardest of hearts soften up and allow the love of forgiveness to heal all pain.

This is a woman who has every reason to harbor bitterness toward a DL man, even though she leaves it unclear whether or not it was the DL man who transmitted HIV to her (and I don't want to assume). Still, she found a way to redeem her tragedy by helping others, liberating herself from useless bitterness, and learning to trust again. She may be unusual in her capacity for forgiveness, but her story shows the powerful liberating effect forgiveness can offer us all.

Dear Mr. King,

    I just wanted to say thank you for the information on your website. I believe my thirty-five-year-old son is a DL brother. He is presently out of town on business. However, on his return I would like to really speak to him about his lifestyle and be sure that he and his girlfriend are protected. I think this will be a nerve-wracking conversation . . . but one that is necessary.

This mother loves her son enough to talk to him about his behavior. I have always said that mothers know. Mothers know when their sons are gay, or when their sons are lying. This mother, who wants to help her son and tell him that she is there for him, is a wonderful example of how one person can help save an innocent person from getting hurt.

Exercising the will necessary for difficult conversations of this sort is one of the hardest things to do, but critically important. But this intuitive mother also touches on another important point: It's not just the role of the spouse to confront the DL man—anyone who knows about it can do so. I'll never forget the story of one DL man whose wife, after she caught him with another man, went to his mother to report her findings. Her mother-in-law just waved her hand and said, "Girl, he's been doing that for a long time now, don't worry about it." If we know a loved one is engaging in this kind of destructive behavior, it makes sense to do what we can to provide an open, nonjudgmental forum for them to unburden themselves.

Dear Mr. King,

I got an e-mail message from a friend of mine about DL brothers and your book coming out. I was more than interested because I think my man may be a DL brother. I hate to think that it might be true, but there are too many things that can't be explained and makes me wonder and worry.

I get HIV tested every six to seven months and I am negative as of right now. I am looking for some answers to my situation and maybe a shoulder to lean on at the same time, because I love him madly and deeply. I am afraid to even approach him with something so horrific. Please help me.

This is a case where it seems like the writer might have reason to believe her man is on the DL. But it's the hardest thing in the world to deal with, because it's simply not something any woman wants to confront in her life. She's doing all the right things, getting tested and trying her best to find a support system that will help her pull through this. But even when we do all the right things, heartbreak can be inevitable. It can also be overcome, so fear of heartbreak should never hold us back from the truth.

If your man loves you as much as you love him, then he will have no problem listening to your concerns. Many DL men love their women. But because they don't understand why they are attracted to men, they live in confusion and fear. Many want to get caught so they can stop living the lie. I would tell any women who is having any concern about her man's behavior to talk to him straight out. If he loves you and is dealing with this issue, it might be something he has been wanting to share with you. You might be that person that can set him free and allow him to be honest with you and either work out your relationship or end it to be with a man.

Dear JL,

I've just found out that my husband has been living his life on the down low. He just recently told me and I am devastated. I am confused as hell because he wants to stay with me, but why on earth would he want me and men too? I never heard of anything like this before. I am completely taken off guard. What is the best way to respond to him? I don't know if my heart can let me or if I should allow him to continue his lifestyle without me.

I applaud this woman's husband for being honest. Now, if you're in a situation like this you have to ask yourself if the love you have for him and the love he has for you is strong enough to help both of you through this process. If you both agree to separate and divorce, you still can be friends and be parents to your children, if there are any. I'd advise this woman to continue to talk about this and seek out professional counseling. You both have made big steps toward the healing process.

Dear Mr. King,

I'm a thirty-six-year-old woman who has actually withdrawn from having sex with men due to the scare of reading topics about the DL. I have not been able to prove this, but my own experience of intimacy with a man who was strongly rumored to have been bisexual scared me to death. This was confirmed by a warning from a hairdresser that said he saw a drag queen getting into his Beamer one evening. Yikes! He has since moved away, which also makes me wonder what the deal is. And the last time I saw him he dropped a lot of weight, which he says had a lot to do with the humid climate where he lives now.

I am completely paranoid about having sex, whether casual or in a serious relationship. I just can't imagine going out like that. No way.

I am crazy about intimacy and sex but feel the risk of getting sick is so not worth it. However, given that a large amount of women contracting the disease happen to be married, it just makes me want to shut down my sexual feelings even more.

Am I crazy? I mean, I have to have sex sometime, and with the summer months approaching, the fine men who do love to pursue women like me will be on the prowl.

Please help.

When I read letters like this, part of me feels like telling my correspondents to be sure they don't let all of the threats out there, including DL men, turn them into celibates. Sex is an important part of life and can be an overwhelmingly positive thing if practiced with care.

But that's really the key: There's no need to rush into it if you're feeling unsure or unsafe. The priority should be in finding someone out there who can be a responsible, healthy sexual partner, rather than just getting it while it's hot.

Dear JL,

I am a female, forty-eight years of age, and enjoyed your book immensely. I finished it just tonight. However, I related to your book on an entirely different level.

I am attracted to bi men. They must be muscular and not gay looking, as you have described the DL man. My attraction is solely in the fantasy stage. I have never acted upon it. I find it very erotic and it is a turn-on for me. I feel compassionate to the DL man because I really know of the drive that consumes them. I have that drive. It is not a bad thing. My fantasy is to watch them. I love strong men. Therefore, I can understand why the down-low man can want them so.

I emphatically agree with you on the point that these sexual

157

encounters should lend consideration to protection because it involves so many other people.

I just wanted to share with you my craving to watch two masculine virile men or maybe participate (not sure of that, but it is a thought).

I'm including this letter because here's a woman unafraid to indulge in boundary-breaking fantasies, but at the same time understands that the first commitment must be to safety. Let's face it, since the beginning of time people have been getting turned on and turned out by all kinds of things, so let's not kid ourselves into thinking this is all brand-new. Many people suppress their sexual fantasies. I have met both men and women who shared with me their fetishes and their "freakiness" that they would never share with anyone, from wanting to spank their man while he is wearing panties to wanting to have sex in public places. Many of us are starved to explore our sexuality. Because people are very judgmental and would think that a woman attracted to bisexual men as sick, many people can only live out their dreams in their minds. I love being free of any binds and hang-ups. Once you taste sexual freedom and you are not breaking the law or hurting anyone, you never want to go back to that kind of bondage.

But while sexual fantasy and experimentation are, of course, fine among consenting adults, no one should ever take sex lightly, for health reasons or just for reasons of our general well-being.

◆◆◆

The voices of these women are a small reflection of the many that are in some way affected by the DL behavior. I am often pained by some of their messages to me. Mostly I am concerned about how uninformed many of these woman are about sexual health. But the encouraging thing is to see that the dialogue is opening up, that people are becoming less afraid to air their thoughts and concerns. And that can only be a good thing.

7

MEN SPEAK OUT

The DL has been more closely associated with men than women, as far as where the guilt lies, which doesn't mean that women aren't out there creeping in lots of different ways. But the DL phenomenon, despite the fact that there are some DL women, is clearly associated with men. In the past year, I have been approached by so many different men with a variety of views on the topic.

The world needs to hear from men on what they feel about sexuality, men on the DL, and how this issue has impacted them and those around them. There are many gay men who have openly expressed how they feel about DL men on websites and at conferences and retreats. I recently spent two days just reading comments that were posted on a popular discussion board about me and the DL topic, and some of the discussions got so hot and there were so many conflicting opinions about men on the DL, that I don't think any of the gay men who were in on the discussion really understood why this was a subject of such importance to women. Most of them wanted to laugh and talk about men on the down low. Many shared their personal stories and some even openly admitted that they were involved with a man who was on the DL. But this is not necessarily a representative view among the gay community.

As for straight men, I have repeatedly challenged them to come forward and let women know that there are 100 percent straight black men who they can date, love, marry, and be sexually involved with. I told a group of my straight friends that instead of keeping quiet and getting upset, you need to be seen and heard. Stand up and let sisters know that you are not confused, that you don't have an interest in having sex with a man, and that you are comfortable with your sexuality. I have asked fathers, brothers, sons, and husbands to think about their female relatives and friends and try to help educate them where the need exists on the importance of safe sex and a safe-sex lifestyle. I told an agitated straight brother in L.A. that I understood why he was upset about so much attention being put on the group of men who are on the DL, and how it is impacting his life, but I also asked him wouldn't he rather know that he informed his daughter about this behavior so that she was aware before she got hurt by not knowing. After a while he understood my point and agreed that even though he wouldn't like being accused, women needed to be able to ask the questions that could help them avoid getting hurt.

I wanted to give men an opportunity to be heard in this

book, so I asked several brothers to speak out about the DL issue. I received input from gay men, straight men, and even men on the DL.

Here is what one had to say:

Dear JL,

I was caught by surprise when I heard about the DL life earlier this year. I have never known gay culture to exist in the comfort of my own middle-class black neighborhood. There were always guys in school people said were gay, either because they talked differently or had a swish in their walk. But that was just grade school talk. After the lightswitch came on in black women everywhere as a result of the *Oprah* show, I noticed that my conversations with women seemed to start with "Are you a down-low brother?" instead of traditional questions like "Do you have a job?" and "Do you still live with your mom?" I can recall being at Max's, one of Houston's top urban spots, and I was talking to a fine black sister about life, politics, and everything in between. Before we traded phone numbers, she asked, "You're not on the DL right?" She said it with a sneer, which suggested she was joking, but the mere fact that she was bold enough to ask me something like that told me that deep inside it truly mattered to her. And though I wanted to be mad at her for calling me out of my comfort zone, deep inside I appreciated her asking me. I am not homophobic, but I am a straight black man. I am twenty-three years old, and for the first time in my life, I had to defend my straightness. I'm sure other brothers can probably relate to a certain degree. Nevertheless, we now have another societal problem to deal with.

But I am not naive. There is something seriously wrong with our culture because we are the ones that have produced these

DL men. We have said, maybe subconsciously, in our church circles, our fraternities and clubs, and the upbringing of a new generation that being gay is not right. Thus these cats are not free to be themselves, causing an even new double-consciousness, something W.E.B. DuBois preached nearly a hundred years ago. Back then it was about being black and American; now it's about black folks loving the same gender. Yet I see it as the same kind of force that rips light and dark black America away from each other. Some dark-skin folks I know feel so self-conscious about their black skin they would even go as far as to bleach themselves to fit the ideal image of beauty. But the only thing that will come as a result of all the skin bleaching (other than looking like a fake-ass Michael Jackson) is an unfulfilled person. I believe DL brothers try so hard to fit into the image of having a wife and kids and the family life that is so promoted by black America, they lose insight into themselves. And like the people not happy inside their skin, this not being fulfilled is why DL brothers stray from their wives and girlfriends and bring diseases back. I may not be the most knowledgeable person on the DL culture because I do not live it, but to all the people who close their minds where the gay life is concerned, look into remedying our problems by not judging folks because they are gay or have AIDS or don't believe what you do. It may be your pastor, your doctor, brother/sister, or friend who is living the DL life. And DL brothers (and sisters too) out there who are still doing the damn thing with both women and men, do me one favor: Just be honest. Don't give all black men a bad rap because of society's values. Go ahead and free yourself.

Frank is a DL man from a large city in the Midwest, and I talked to him to try to get the active DL man's perspective on things. I'm not going to add too much commentary to my recounting of what he said: You can just read it and make your own conclusions.

Many DL men feel that when they have sex with a man they are not cheating. Frank told me that he doesn't cheat on his woman with other women. He said that his girl satisfies his sexual need for woman, so he never cheats with women. He told me that he wanted to tell his woman that he was on the DL, but he didn't because of the possibility of her not understanding and leaving, which is not worth the gamble. Plus, he told me he loved her with all his heart and didn't want to lose her.

He told me that many of his DL friends are okay with playing the field and sleeping with different men all the time, but couldn't see themselves being in a committed relationship with a man.

I asked him about the difference between sex with men and women—if a woman was satisfying him sexually, at least to some extent, why did he feel the need to go out and have sex with men, too. He said that sex with a man is very fulfilling in a very different way that's hard to explain in words. He said at its best it just comes naturally to him, just like when he is making love to his woman.

He is one DL brother who doesn't plan on telling his woman. As long as he can keep his two separate lives, then he will. But he wants to find one brother who he can develop a relationship with and just be with that one man, while also staying with his woman. It would be perfect, he told me, if he had a male sexual partner who was also the sort of friend he could invite home for dinner and have him get to know his wife. That way he wouldn't have to feel as if he was sneaking all the time and always away from the house. If he had a friend who he was sexually involved with, then he would bring him home and could even call his woman and tell her where he was without raising any concerns.

He always uses condoms when he is screwing men, and when he is with a man, he makes sure that they know he is not going to put himself or his family at risk to get a disease.

The final man's voice I'm going to give you is that of Tracy J. Sipp, author of *The Cry of the Little Boy—Overcoming the Struggle*. Tracy speaks from a religious perspective but has something to say to even those of us who are not believers. His main point echoes that of the first brother in the chapter: that we all have to open our arms with love and understanding to each and every member of the community. It's that kind of love that will finally put an end to the DL lifestyle.

There are those who cheer the bashing of God's children—those children who struggle with the fight against the spirit of homosexuality. Ignorance has always been an easy excuse for them to target the homosexual, but God encourages us to read and study the Bible (his word) in order to learn to accept those individuals who are struggling with personal demons. It is especially the responsibility of those who have been chosen to pastor or minister or lead others not to stand before their congregations and belittle those struggling with homosexuality in particular. God sees us all the same, and therefore does not see one sin as being more deplorable than another. To God sin is sin.

Indeed, the spirit of homosexuality is an abomination to God. However, please keep in mind that it is a spirit like any other sinful spirit that the Body of Christ faces. We, like God, should hate all sin, and hating the sinfulness of homosexuality should be no different. However to have a personal hate against those struggling with the spirit of homosexuality is just as sinful in God's eyes. Passing judgment to those in the Body of Christ struggling with homosexuality is wrong, and God isn't pleased with so-called Christians who sit in judgment of others. The Bible shows us time and time again that God takes no pleasure in those who inflict personal attacks on individuals struggling with homosexuality; using derogatory and inflammatory names against them such as *faggot* is not biblical! The term *homosexual* is the correct biblical name for one who involves themselves sexually with the same gender.

Because homosexuality is a sin that most churches can't or don't deal with, some church folk believe names like *faggot* and other such names are fine to use, because the spirit of homosexuality is depicted in the Bible as a sin offensive to God. However, the dictionary sites the word *faggot* as "a name used disparagingly against a male homosexual." The word *disparage* means: degrade, below one's class; lower in rank or reputation; depreciate by indirect means; and speak slightingly about. Our God would not condone this kind of demeaning reference to a soul. The word *faggot* and other words such as *sissy* and *punk* are words used to continue to belittle homosexuals in the way that nigger is meant to demean the African American. These are very hateful words that God is not pleased with.

Christians are taught to reach others through *love*, especially those who have been called as leaders to the ministry. In order to help those struggling to be delivered from any sin or sinful lifestyle, we as Christians are to continue to seek God's direction so that we might become better Christians more pleasing in God's sight. Because we all battle sin, there is no one group of people who is better than another. We are all in a spiritual battle against the sins of the enemy. Since the beginning of Christianity judgmental churchgoers within the Body of Christ have always been taught that the spirit of homosexuality is beneath all other sin. Some consider homosexuals as a group of weak individuals who want to be something other than what God has made them. This is where the ignorance begins. Let's be clear, all homosexuals do not desire to be females, and surely all homosexuals are not sexual predators preying on men or boys because of an uncontrollable sexual perversion.

It is very important to create a dialogue about the spirit of homosexuality, especially within the church. Please keep in mind that the spirit of homosexuality is a spirit like all other sin, and the Body of Christ must begin to understand that those with this spirit are in a spiritual warfare.

Everything begins with education, and it is the obligation of the spiritual leaders to help teach their members the truth about the spirit of homosexuality since hatred is being generated within the church because of ignorance. It is shameful that the church is still hiding and is not allowing the Body of Christ to get to the root of this demonic spirit called homosexuality. While ignorance within the church in this area is still allowed, we are losing thousands of souls to death because this topic is not acceptable to talk about in the house of God. Because pastors and other spiritual leaders are still unwilling to learn how this spirit affects so many souls, we will always have a hell-bound group of individuals searching for freedom and feeling worthless by living a life away from God's will. By continuing to avoid this issue and allowing the ignorance of this spirit to remain, many innocent individuals including their family members continue to suffer.

It is disheartening to think that homosexuals are the only group of people who are never expected to discuss their struggles, hurts, or pains, because heterosexuals are not open to hearing about their life challenges. Other types of addictions are real enough and acceptable to the heterosexual including addictions to drugs, heterosexual sex, alcohol, prostitution, pimping, and others. It has become part of our culture to provide addiction programs that help recovering addicts in these areas, but in all this time there still remains little help or acceptance for the homosexual. When discussing homosexuality, it is clear to see that it is the only form of addiction that does not receive the same compassion that is extended to others.

It has been said by some ministers, pastors, and spiritual leaders that those struggling with the spirit of homosexuality should not be allowed to function in key leadership positions in the church. My question to them is this: Should Christians struggling with other sinful spirits be allowed to be used by God? If not, then who would be left to do the work within the Body of Christ? No one is perfect enough to throw the first stone.

In reading the Bible one learns that many prophets and other significant individuals struggled with sinful behaviors and still went on to be very powerful representatives for God. Although these biblical figures struggled with their personal sins everyday, God never turned his back on them in the way many Christians do today. One must know that the Holy Spirit chooses to use whomever He pleases; no human being is in control of who the Holy Spirit chooses to use.

Remember God is the judge and jury, and thank God that he opens up his arms to all who should receive Jesus Christ. I encourage you to be like God. Open up your arms to those who are struggling to live with personal demons, don't judge but pray for them, because until we can learn to love and pray sincerely for others, humanity as a whole will continue to suffer and God Almighty will continue to turn his face away from us. Love covers a multitude of sins; God said it . . . if only we could take the time to practice it!!! May God Bless You.

8

TO THINE OWN SELF
BE TRUE

Since my book was released, I have had an opportunity to repair the relationships within my family. When I was invited to be a guest on *Oprah*, I
asked my daughter, Ebony, to join me and be there in the
audience as my support system. At dinner the evening
before the show she and I had a wonderful, open conversation. I told her to ask me anything that she wanted to and I
would respect her as an adult and honestly share with her. It
was definitely not your conventional father-daughter conversation, but it was one that made us both feel better. We
laughed a lot that night. After dinner I suggested that she
read the galley copy of my book. It was incredible for me to
be able to share with her a part of my life that had been a
secret for so long. Too long.

I had the chance to explain to her that she was one of
the main reasons for me eventually spreading the message
about the DL. As a father, I know the responsibility I have to

protect her. I am more than aware of the growing DL community, and when I thought about Ebony, my cousins, nieces, and all the other women who could be having sex with men who were not telling them about their double life, I knew that I had to expose this unsafe lifestyle. I do not want my daughter, or any other woman, to get infected with HIV or any kind of STD from a man who lies to her about his down-low lifestyle. I also have her emotional state to consider. The pain this kind of deceipt causes is unfair. No woman should have to go through that.

Fortunately my exwife is my friend. We have always had a healthy relationship, and I was happy to hear that she was going to share her story for other women to understand. She wants to show them that they can survive and still maintain a healthy relationship with men who live this life. She also wants to explain to the women that there is a way to reach out to that man who is ready to come clean with his story. I still go to her for support, we are still parents to our children, and one day we will be grandparents to our grandchildren. My having been on the DL will not stop that. My three adult children are still there for me and support me in all that I do, as I support them. We are closer today then we have ever been. That is a benefit of being free and not having to lie about who you are, who you love, or who you date. Life is too short.

My father and I had a big strain in our relationship for some time. I am happy to say that things are wonderful between us now. We have a stronger respect for each other. I respect him as the man who raised me and my brother to be men who have never been in trouble for any crime, strung out on drugs, or neglectful to our children. He was a wonderful role model, and I love him for always being there for us. He is a very loving eighty-six-year-old man, father, and grandfather, and is very active in his church.

Does he know all the details of my sexual life? Probably not. My sexuality is not important in our relationship. I didn't have conversations about it when I was twenty-one, I am sure not going to do it now. He doesn't care about it. I am his son. We have gotten so close since the book came out, not because he read and understood it (he didn't), but because now that my story is out, I am no longer uncomfortable around him. I don't have to lie just to keep him happy. Ironically, by talking so much about my sex life, I've come to realize more than ever that there is more to me than just my sexuality. My father acknowledges those things and that is what we focus on. He only asks if I'm happy and if I'm taking care of myself. He wants to know if I am going to church and paying my tithes. That is what is important to him.

There were a few occasions where people from his community or his church have called him to tell him that they read my book and ask him what he thinks of it. Many, including relatives, have done that out of hate or jealousy of my success. Since they can't get to me, they have tried to hurt him. I don't want him to have to deal with that. He is a happy senior citizen who is living a wonderful life. He has ignored them and never once mentioned or questioned me about it. At this point in our relationship, I don't need him to change his beliefs. I don't take offense to the fact that he believes homosexuality is a sin. He has stopped preaching to me. And out of respect I don't force my sexuality on him.

The fact is, I have changed. I think the biggest change is that I now have a freedom to be whoever I want to be. I no longer have to worry about being judged, because I am comfortable with who I am. I am a bisexual man who no longer has to hide his sexuality. I used to be on the down low. I used to lie about my sexuality when someone would ask me. I used to put all the women that I was with after my divorce at risk and cause emotional damage. I used to hate to look at myself in the mirror. When I divorced, I moved out of my hometown, where my wife and I had lived and raised our kids, where I had gone to church, socialized with the community, and worked. I moved and started another life. I dated women and even got engaged to three other women while I continued to have sex with other men. I was unable to see the path of pain I was creating for these women, even when they would look me in my eyes and tell me that they loved me. I was unable to stop the behavior.

I did not practice this behavior intending to hurt anyone. I was clearly confused. I knew that I had feelings for men even when my family was pressuring me to bring a wife home. I knew it when they would casually bring up kids and grandkids. These are normal requests from family members when dealing with a man that is not confused about his sexuality. But no matter what kind of subtle or not-so-subtle pressure I got to settle down into a "normal" life, I never could. Not until now.

My life has become a true picture of what an open bisexual life can be about. I don't have to cover up who I am with. I am also free when it comes to being with a woman. I can now be honest with her. I am not deceiving anyone anymore. I was on a date with a female about a month ago. We were out dancing and having a great time. A good-looking brother walked in and she noticed me checking him out. We both laughed because she also thought he was good-looking. She actually told me at the end of the night that she appreciated my honesty. You can't imagine how free I felt. I was no longer causing pain and at the same time I am free to be me. I believe that a lot of women are cool with my lifestyle as long as they are given the truth and a choice.

I used to have this overwhelming urge for fast, easy, unemotional sex, but it was always followed by guilt and denial. I was afraid to be with a man physically and actually have my mind and heart there, too. It was like I couldn't give my mind or heart to another man. It seemed that since I was young I was told that that kind of connection was saved for a husband and wife, not two men lusting after each other. Because now I accept who I am, I can love and be with a man the same way that I can love and be with a woman.

One of the most rewarding moments of my life was when I was able to take home a brother who I was involved with to meet my father. I had to visit my father one weekend and decided that I wanted him to meet this brother. I didn't want to go alone, and I didn't want to have him sit at a restaurant while I visited with my father. I was tired of lying to my dad and telling him that I was dating a female when I wasn't. I had been on every television network, in every major newspaper, on the cover of *Jet* magazine, and had written a national bestseller, all representative of my former DL lifestyle. The irony is that with all that exposure, my father still to this day has no idea what all the hype is about or even that I am attached to it. Every now and then someone from my old hometown will tell me that they tried to tell my father what I was up to. I always wonder to myself, why? Why try to bring all of this drama to an eighty-three-year-old old-school man from Alabama who has gotten this far in life with a fourth-grade education and his faith? But they always tell me my father's reaction and it's always the same: "Praise the Lord." Luckily, at this point in his life, he's found a peaceful place and he's staying there.

As my friend and I drove through my small hometown, I reflected back on how far my life has come. I remembered the first time I spoke in front of a large crowd of people and told my personal story of when I was living on the DL, how my palms sweated and I had to fight down the urge to lie and dissemble in the way I'd trained myself to do whenever talking about the personal details of my life. I thought about how much my life has changed over the past year, and about all the many roads I have traveled to get to be the man I am today.

As we pulled up in front of my dad's house, I didn't feel the fear that I once felt when I would go to my parents' house. I looked at my partner and told him, "It's going to be okay." He knew that this was a big step for me. To take a man home was not something that I had ever done. I thought that my dad would be able to tell just by looking at my friends if they were gay. He had always been so negative about gay men. I can still hear the comments he made when I was a child about openly gay men at the church we attended or his very strong opinion about men on television who were gay. If they were a little on the fem side he would make a comment that those men were "queer" and that God didn't approve of homosexuality. I always made sure that everything I did would appear to my dad as 100 percent heterosexual, and that I never gave him anything to be concerned about. Even today, as a grown adult with adult children, I was still worrying about what he would think about my friend, and if it would make him think that I was gay. That was funny. Mr. Down Low to the world and the world knows everything about my sex life, past and present, and I was sweating that by taking my friend inside my dad's house would cause me to lose favor in his eyes.

We got out of the car and walked up the steps to the front porch. I opened the door since he never locked the screen door, and he was sitting in his favorite chair in the living room. My mom, who had passed away in 2002, still left a strong presence inside the house. I could see her sitting in the kitchen drinking a cup of tea. I could smell her cooking my favorite foods—macaroni and cheese, collard greens, sweet potatoes, and her famous bread dressing. I miss her, and every time I walk into my parents' house, it takes me a moment or two to regroup and realize that she is not there in physical form, only in spirit.

As I walked into the living room, I bent over and hugged my dad. We had started hugging each other only recently. As he has gotten older, he has become more open to hugs from me. Having him hug me was something I loved, and I wished that he had hugged me as a child growing up. But he never did. Now I enjoyed it. I introduced him to my friend, and he reached out and shook his hand. My friend told my father that he had heard a lot about him, and that he was ready for the "sermon" that my dad gave every-body who came to the house. My father started laughing and told my friend that he would get a word from God before he left the house. We all laughed and that broke the ice.

I had briefed my friend on how he could get to my dad next. I needed him to win him over right away. I told him to be himself and that to remember that my dad had been a deacon at his church for more than fifty years and he loved his church. So if my friend talked about how good God is, and how he loved going to church, that would keep my dad's mind away from any thoughts about us having sex or being in a relationship. Strange but true. I know my dad, and I know what would make him feel comfortable with me bringing a man home. It had been awhile since I had brought any women home, and I'm sure he had thought about that; every now and again he would ask me when I was going to bring a sister home. The truth is, he was not in touch with who I am as a bisexual man, at least not in detail, since we never sat down and had a heart-to-heart talk about it. I really don't think he knows anything about my fame and reputation as the down-low expert. People find that hard to believe, but it is true. He has never asked me about my book, nor has he ever asked me anything about the down-low issue. Not one word.

I brought him a picture of me and Oprah, which I had asked her to take with me after the show. I had had it framed and I wanted my father to have it. It's a big picture and he put it on top of the television in the living room with other family pictures. He loved Oprah and asked me how I knew her. He said, "You must be somebody important if you know Oprah." That was all he said, not another word. I feel that until he asks me about my work, the book, or my new sexual freedom, then I will not bring it up. He is an eighty-three-year-old man who is enjoying his life, and I don't feel the need to rock his world about my coming to acceptance of who I am. I am his son, I am responsible, and I make sure that my dad hears from me on weekly basis, and as long as he knows that I am not starving, homeless, or broke, he is happy.

This is exactly the kind of thing that divides gay and bisexual people from different cultural backgrounds. Many black gay and bisexual men feel that there sexual lives is their business alone, which, at its worst, leads to DL behavior and contributes to a culture of silence around issues of sexuality. But it's still okay, I believe, to show discretion in life. My sexuality is not a weapon that I want to use to antagonize my father in his sunset years. As long as I'm out with those I'm intimate with and clear with myself, then I think I'm doing my duty to both the people I love and to my own sense of self.

At the end of that visit, I felt so good about me. I was able to have my friend with me and enjoy the day with my dad. And my dad, my friend, and I all had a wonderful visit. It had nothing to do with anything but a dad and a son spending the day together. The lesson that I learned that day was that I had spent the majority of my life trying to keep up a front of being overly masculine to please my dad, and that I had not allowed him or my mother to get to know the real me. And that was because I didn't know me.

This newfound freedom and self-acceptance is something that I wish I had years ago. If I had not lived in fear of what others thought about me, or worried about if my parents would have stopped loving me, or that God would put me in hell, I feel that I would have had a different life. Maybe I would not have lied to so many women, maybe I would have turned out a different person, maybe my journey would have taken me down a path where I could have been the first man in my small hometown to pave the way for other men who were confused about their sexuality and had no role model to follow. Maybe I could have been the one person that could have broken the tradition that allowed my pastor to preach hatred against gay members to the point where his words planted seeds of fear in my young life and I'm sure in the minds of other young men in our church who were just like me. Then again, maybe my life was shaped the way it was so I could do the work I am doing today.

I have learned so much about people over the course of the past year. I have experienced hatred that I could never understand. I have had to debate about my personal story, a life that I lived many years ago, and turn around and question myself to confirm that what I was saying was true. I have had to explain to friends and family members that I am not crazy, that I am doing what I'm doing because I'm convinced it *is* the right thing. I have had to argue with people who have accused me of making money off HIV and said that everything I did and continue to do is motivated by money. I have cried myself to sleep when I wanted it all to go away. And I have celebrated my success with people who understand me and lift me up.

I have faced the person that I look at in the mirror every day and learned to love him. I have prayed to my God and have received His word that He has my back and will never let me fail.

One of my favorite songs is "When You've Been Blessed" by Ms. Patti LaBelle. The song says that when God gives you more than others, you should pass it on. When you have been blessed, you don't keep it, you pass it on. I have adopted that song as my song. I have made that song the song that motivates me to give back to my community from all the blessings that I have received. I established the Lillie Mae King Foundation in 2004, named in honor of my mother as a way to give back. I personally fund the foundation and the foundation has three areas that we fund: African American youth, African American MSM, and neglected dogs. My mother loved dogs and would treat them as members of her own family. So the foundation will provide funding for organizations that take in stray dogs and train them as pets for people who are suffering from AIDS and in hospice houses. We all have to do our part and bring a change so that we can eliminate HIV and relationship and social issues (homophobia) in the world.

But more than that, even, my true blessing comes from the feedback I get from people who have responded to this message. The responses are not always picture-perfect, because life isn't always picture-perfect. But they're real and show that the message has gotten out.

I recently sat down with a brother in St. Louis who is living on the down low. He and I talked for hours about what he was doing and I tried to convince him to come clean to his wife and to seriously consider the possibility that he might have to go on without her. He told me that he loved her too much to leave her, that he couldn't leave her, but that he also wanted to stop his behavior but couldn't. He shared with me that he had tried in the past to stop the desire, but he had lost the struggle every time. He asked me how I did it. He wanted to know what was the pivotal point in my life that made me stop living a lie, and how was I able to keep my head up and maintain a healthy and loving relationship with my children. I told him that once I learned to love myself, it was easy for others to love me. I let him know it wasn't exactly easy, and that the journey has not been smooth. But in the end it worked out for the best. I told him that he might have to take a beating, but in the long run, he will be a better person, and the people in his life will be better off. He took my advice and told me he would pray over it, and then he thanked me for being a role model for himself and other men who are still living on the down low. The idea that my messed-up life and the trials I've gone through might give some guidance to another man in the same situation is an ample reward.

On the other hand, I sometimes get feedback that is downright vicious. I received an e-mail from a sister who called me every ugly name in the book. She wrote that I had divided the community and set back black relationships. She went on to say that she didn't believe anything that I wrote in my first book, that she was not going to stop having sex, and what she did with her body was her business, so I could kiss her ass. She ended her e-mail with this statement, which was typed in a large bold underlined font: **<u>I hope you die of HIV.</u>** At first I was upset and wanted to e-mail her and ask her what I did to her, why would she say these hurtful things to me, and what could I do or say to get her to like me. Of course, it's this same instinct to please (and to feel shame) that keeps so many brothers in the closet or on the DL. Then I remembered what a very close friend who is also in the public eye said to me. That no matter what you do or say, you can't possibly please everyone. If you give all of your money away, people will talk about you. If you keep it, they will talk about you. If you tell them what they want to hear, they will turn on you, and if you don't tell them what they want to hear, they will turn on you. All you can do is stay true to your word and continue to walk the path that you are on. Keep good people around you and don't read anything nonconstructively negative that is written or said about you. All that will do is steal your joy and eat you alive. I have kept those words in my mind, and when I get these sorts of messages, they no longer have the same impact on my life.

The same day I received that nasty e-mail, I got an e-mail from another woman telling me that my book had opened up her eyes and forced her to look at her past and current behavior. She shared with me that she has had sex with many men, just to feel needed and wanted, and she never asked about their status, if they were gay, bisexual, or anything. She just wanted them to show her some attention and some love. She needed to be held and she loved being loved by a strong black man. She wrote that even when she got a small STD that was cured by taking a few pills, that didn't inspire her to take control of her body. Even when she overheard one of her exboyfriends on the phone talking to someone about meeting them later, she kept blinders on so she would not get hurt. She allowed men to use her for whatever reason they wanted. As long as they told her they loved her, she was happy. After she read my book, she said it was like the blinders were taken off, and she saw what she had become: a women who had given up her life to men, just so she could feel needed and loved, when in reality it was all fake and make believe. She said in her e-mail that my book is on her nightstand, and every time the urge comes over her to call one of the men who've done her dirt, she looks at my picture and talks to me about what she is feeling and, as crazy as this sounds, she told me that I talk back to her. She told me that she and I have had many long conversations, and I have talked her out of giving up her body just to feel wanted. She also told me that she would always be thankful for me being in her life, even though we have never met.

This e-mail really cut to the heart of what drives not just the DL phenomenon, but so many dysfunctional sexual practices. In the black community, like many other communities, there is a sense that because we have these major institutions—the church, the historically black colleges, fraternities and sororities, and so on—that we're automatically going to feel embraced by others. But the truth is different. Many of us, despite the surface of community, are terribly alone. In spite of all the ways we connect to each other—from the church to the nightclub—there's something deeper that's missing in our lives. It's this hole that drives us into dangerous sexual behavior as a way of avoiding the pain of dealing with the truth about ourselves and the sometimes crushing loneliness that we can feel.

If that's the problem, what's the solution? It's easy and hard: We have to love each other more. We have to create safe places for each other and reach out to each other when we're struggling. We have to go beyond the surface of community and love and actually start practicing it. In my conversations with hundreds of people dealing with the DL problem from every angle, that's the truth that comes out again and again: These are people who are desperate for love, for forgiveness, and for acceptance.

When I read these types of e-mail, I know what I have done is the right thing. I know that I have to learn to deal with the bitter as well as the sweet. But if I continue to allow God to use me, he will keep me protected and he will order my steps. For this year, my scriptural affirmation is: *No weapon formed against me shall prosper.*

I wrote in my first book that I am not the authority about the DL behavior, that others would come forward and claim to be the expert, the professional, and challenge me and my opinion. And that has and is happening; many who are motivated by jealousy and envy of my success. You have to remember that I didn't want to write a book in the first place. I wrote it because I was asked to write one. When I wrote it, I went into the process unprepared and unaware. Naive. I thought everyone would love and support me and sing my praises. But if you put yourself out there, you open yourself up to criticism. And I wasn't ready. I wasn't ready to see friends turn on me or people pushed out to discredit me. I've told people at my readings: I'm not a healthcare professional and you shouldn't read my book as a medical journal. But at the same time my message is clear and true. I've created a movement of awareness—that was my purpose from day one. I wanted to write a book that would speak to this crucial issue to and write it in a way that it could be read by everyday folks—from Shanana to Dr. Shanana, as I told my editor. And they've all read it or heard about it now, and we're now, as a community, facing up to some important truths.

When my daughter and exwife and I were together recently, it felt so good to see the look on my daughter's face to see her parents talking and laughing. There was no anger, pain, hurt, or lies. We were a family that has survived some hard times. But we'd gotten through them. I was talking to my exwife about my book tour, and she and my daughter were most interested in making sure that I was taking care of myself. They both could care less about all the DL business; they had gotten over it and past it. The most important thing to them was that I was happy and healthy. And that's what we're going to do as a community. We'll get over and past the DL and all of these issues of sexual confusion and concern, and we'll pull together, making sure that we're all healthy and happy.

ACKNOWLEDGMENTS

I want to give a special thank-you to the following people who are part of my inner circle. You keep me grounded and provide the strength to be J.L.:

Ebony M. King. My beautiful daughter, who is the only woman in my life. I love you. Everything I do is for you.

James Brandon King. My "look-alike" son, who I am so proud of. I love you more than life.

Anthony D. King. You have become the perfect role model for young fathers. You live for your family, and it shows.

My dad, Louis V. King. Thank you for always loving me and telling me to keep God first. I am happy that Ms. Ellis is in your life and I thank her for making you smile.

Acknowledgments

I am a bestselling author only because of the following: Oprah Winfrey. No more needs to be said, except she is truly a gift from God.

Bookstores—especially black owned and operated—that made sure my first book, *On the Down Low,* was front and center and invited me for book signings.

Radio and TV talk shows that featured me and my book.

The black book clubs who chose my book as a selection of the month. You are the lifeline of black authors.

The African American female organizations that invited me to speak at their events, especially the Delta Sigma Theta Sorority, Inc.

The numerous magazines, newspapers, online newsletters, TV stations, and any and all print media who covered me and my work, especially *Jet*, *Ebony*, *Essence*, *Rolling Out*, and *A&U*.

A very special thank-you to each of you who have always been there for me:
Margena A. Christian, Cheryl Burton, Debra Brown, Art "Chat" Sims, D. Jenkins, Anthony Hardaway, Roderick Smith, Marshall Douglas, Denise Jones, Angela Kenyetta, Dr. Ron Simmons, Brenda Browder, the Stone family, Angie Tolliver, and about a hundred others. You know who you are and how special you are to me.

I also thank:

My editor, Chris Jackson, for his amazing skills, and the rest of the Crown team; my co-writer Courtney, the coolest sister I know; and my super agent, Ian Kleinart.

And last, but always first in my life:

Jesus Christ, all praises to You. I love You and acknowledge that everything in my life is according to Your will for me.

ABOUT THE AUTHORS

J. L. King is an HIV/STD prevention activist and author of the bestselling *On the Down Low: A Journey into the Lives of "Straight" Black Men Who Sleep with Men*. His expertise has been cited in national publications such as the *New York Times* and *Essence,* and his television appearances have ranged from *The Oprah Winfrey Show* to Black Entertainment Television (BET). The father of three, he divides his time between Chicago and Atlanta. Visit his website at www.jlking.net.

Courtney Carreras, a freelance writer, is the former editor-in-chief of *YRB* magazine and the author of *The White Man's Guide to Hip Hop Survival*. She lives in Harlem, New York.